Principles of Oral and Maxillofacial Surgery

Fifth edition

Edited by

U. J. Moore

FDSRCS (Eng), PhD (Ncle)
Lecturer in Oral and Maxillofacial Surgery
University of Newcastle-upon-Tyne

b
**Blackwell
Science**

Editorial offices:
Blackwell Science Ltd, 9600 Garsington Road, Oxford OX4 2DQ, UK
    Tel: +44 (0) 1865 776868
Blackwell Publishing Inc., 350 Main Street, Malden, MA 02148-5020, USA
    Tel: +1 781 388 8250
Blackwell Science Asia Pty, 550 Swanston Street, Carlton, Victoria 3053, Australia
    Tel: +61 (0)3 8359 1011

First edition published 1965 by Pergamon Press Ltd as *Principles of Oral Surgery*
Second edition published 1981; Third edition published 1984; Fourth edition published 1991,
    all by Manchester University Press
Fifth edition published by Blackwell Science Ltd 2001
Reprinted 2002, 2006

ISBN-10: 0-632-05438-7
ISBN-13: 978-0-632-05438-1

Library of Congress Cataloging-in-Publication Data

Principles of oral and maxillofacial surgery /
    edited by U.J. Moore.—5th ed.
        p.   cm.
    Includes bibliographical references and index.
    ISBN 0-632-05438-7
    1. Mouth—Surgery.   2. Maxilla—Surgery.
  3. Face—Surgery.   I. Moore, U.J. (Undrell J.)

    RK529.P752 2001
    617.5'2059—dc21   2001018129

A catalogue record for this title is available from the British Library

Set in 10 on 12.5 pt Times
by Best-set Typesetter Ltd, Hong Kong
Printed and bound by Replika Press Pvt. Ltd, India

For further information on Blackwell Publishing, visit our website:
www.blackwellpublishing.com

Principles of Oral and Maxillofacial Surgery

18 AUG

14.

30. N

20. OCT

Contents

Preface to Fifth Edition

Much has been said about the fragmentation of this speciality but this book attempts to broaden its scope to include the established pattern of maxillofacial surgery within the essential roots of undergraduate dental education.

This has been made easier by the excellence of the original text which has been interfered with as little as possible, although the topics of oral cancer, oral and maxillofacial trauma, salivary gland disease, infection, facial deformity and pharmacology have been considerably updated.

Explanation of principles has remained the priority and this is still intended as an undergraduate and early postgraduate text.

Acknowledgements

This textbook had its inception in the early days of the speciality and much has changed within both the discipline and the book since then. It is important to acknowledge those who created the environment for these changes and influenced the contributions to this revised edition.

I am grateful to Professor Peter Thomson who encouraged my desire to see this volume back in print, and to Manchester University Press who generously gave us copyright of the original text. Blackwell Science have willingly accepted the challenge of publishing a new fifth edition with all the revision and inclusion of new material this has involved, and Richard Miles in particular has shown great forbearance and provided much-needed advice.

The VU Press in Amsterdam have generously allowed the reproduction of several illustrations for the chapter on facial deformity.

Even in these days of desktop publishing, secretarial support is important and the contributors would like to thank Mrs Beryl Leggatt for her help.

Finally I would like to thank my father for all he has given, both professionally and personally.

Foreword to the First Edition

There is an increasing need for trained oral surgeons in the world today. An operative field that was a no-man's-land partly controlled by the general surgeon, partly controlled by the dental surgeon, has now come to be the field of a specialised branch of dentistry.

In the past we have had to use books written and published in America, and, fine though these books are, it is refreshing to find a book produced by a British oral surgeon, because in the world today, British oral surgery has undoubtedly the highest general level of training and achievement in the oral surgical field.

Mr J. R. Moore has had considerable practical experience as an oral surgeon in a consultative capacity before devoting his talents to teaching, and he has produced a book of great practical use both to the student or trainee learning oral surgery and also a book of great interest to the established specialist.

I deplore the fragmentation of the dental profession by dividing it into so many specialities, but in the field of oral surgery there are procedures which the dental surgeon would not wish to carry out. Therefore a knowledge of the difficulties and hazards of an oral surgical procedure is essential for the general dental surgeon, who should include this book in his library.

It is with great pleasure that I commend this work of Mr J. R. Moore of University College Hospital to the profession.

T. G. Ward

List of Contributors

J. G. Cowpe
PhD, BDS, FDSRCS (Ed), FDSRCS (Eng)
Professor of Oral Surgery, University of Bristol.

J. G. Meechan
BSc, BDS, PhD, FDSRCPS (Glas)
Senior Lecturer in Oral and Maxillofacial Surgery, University of Newcastle-upon-Tyne.

K. R. Postlethwaite
FRCS, FDSRCS, MBChB, BDS
Consultant in Oral and Maxillofacial Surgery, Royal Victoria Hospitals Trust, Newcastle-upon-Tyne.

P. J. Thomson
BDS, MBBS, MSc, PhD, FDSRCS, FRCS (Ed)
Professor of Oral and Maxillofacial Surgery, University of Newcastle-upon-Tyne.

Chapter 1
The New Patient

- History
- Examination
- Special investigation
- Diagnosis
- Treatment plan

It is difficult to overstress the importance of a good history and thorough clinical examination for every patient. On this the diagnosis is made and the treatment plan based. A full, clearly written record of the original consultation is essential to assess progress following treatment. Particularly is this true if a colleague should be called to see the patient in the practitioner's absence. The medicolegal importance of accurate records cannot be overemphasised.

In hospital and specialist practice this procedure can seldom be relaxed, but the student and the busy practitioner may find it irksome to maintain a high standard when faced with a series of apparently straightforward dental conditions. Nevertheless, sufficient time must be allowed for an unhurried consultation at the first visit. This will help to avoid errors of omission, and may contribute much to the success of treatment and to the interest of the practitioner. With experience, only important facts need be noted, the dental surgeon considering and setting aside the irrelevant points. This technique can be used with safety only after a long apprenticeship during which many histories and examinations have been methodically completed and all the information recorded. In this chapter a system for interviewing and examining patients, and recording findings, is briefly suggested.

History

At the first meeting it is important for the clinician to establish a relationship with the patient and to assess his attitude to the clinical situation. He is seated comfortably and addressed by his name and correct title. The general details of age, sex, marital status, occupation and address together with the names of his

1

general medical and dental practitioner are entered in the notes. At this stage it should be possible to determine whether the patient is anxious or relaxed. The history is then recorded under the headings shown in italics.

The patient will seldom tell his story well. Some will be verbose, others reticent, while the sequence is usually in inverse chronological order with the most recent events first. The art of the good history lies in avoiding leading questions, in eliciting all the essentials, in censoring verbosity and in arranging the facts in their true order, so that the written record is short and logical. Allowing the patient initially to give the history and subsequently writing notes in chronological order whilst rechecking the facts verbally, helps the clinician obtain a concise and accurate account of the patient's symptoms.

Patient referred by

The name and professional status of the person referring is noted.

Complains of (CO)

The patient's chief complaint told *in his own words*. Opinions, professional and otherwise, repeated in an effort to help must be gently set aside and the patient encouraged to describe the symptoms he wants cured, and not his views on the diagnosis.

History of present complaint (HPC)

This is an account *in chronological order* of the disease. When and how it first started, the suspected cause, any exciting factors, and the character of the local lesion such as pain, swelling and discharge. This includes remissions and the effects of any treatment received. General symptoms such as fever, malaise and nausea are also noted.

Previous dental history (PDH)

This records how regularly the patient attends for dental care and the importance he attaches to his teeth. Any past experience of oral surgery is included especially where difficulty occurred in the administration of anaesthetics, the extraction of teeth and the control of bleeding.

Medical history (MH)

A summary in chronological order of the patient's past illnesses. Details of prolonged illness, or those requiring hospital admission or current medication are recorded. The surgeon should exert his critical faculty and write down only those conditions that may affect the diagnosis or treatment. The more important of these medical conditions are discussed in Chapter 3.

The family history (FH)

Occasionally this is of importance in oral surgery. Hereditary diseases such as haemophilia and partial anodontia may be relevant in management of the patient.

The social history (SH)

This includes a brief comment on the patient's occupation and social habits such as exercise, smoking and drinking. The home circumstances are important when surgery is to be performed – that is, whether the patient has far to travel, lives alone or has someone to look after him. These factors may influence the decision to treat him as an in- or out-patient.

Principles of examination

Superficially the dental surgeon's examination may seem very different from that of his medical colleagues, yet the basic principles are the same. It should be made according to a definite system which in time becomes a ritual. In this way errors of omission are avoided.

From the moment the patient enters the surgery he should be carefully observed for signs of physical or of psychological disease which may show in the gait, the carriage, the general manner, or the relationship between parent and child. Too little time is often spent on visual inspection, both intra- and extraorally. Eyes first, then hands, should be the rule, not both together.

In palpation all movements are purposeful and logical, and the touch firm but gentle. The tips of the fingers are used first to locate anatomical landmarks and then to determine the characteristics of the pathological condition. The patient's co-operation is sought so that areas of tenderness may be recognised and the minimum discomfort caused. Wherever possible the normal side is examined simultaneously. Only by such comparison can minor degrees of asymmetry be detected. Swellings situated in the floor of the mouth or in the cheek are felt bimanually with one hand placed in, and one outside, the mouth. Both positive and negative findings are written down as later one may wish to check that at the first visit no abnormality was found in certain structures.

Systematic procedure for examination of the mouth

Extraoral examination

This commences with a general inspection, and palpation of the face including the mandible, maxillary and malar bones, noting the presence of any abnormality such as asymmetry or paralysis of the facial muscles. The eyes, their movements and pupil reactions, are observed together with any difficulty in breathing.

The temporomandibular joints

With the surgeon standing behind the patient, the site of the condyles are identified by palpation whilst the patient opens and closes their mouth.

The joints are examined for tenderness and clicking or crepitus on opening and closing. The range of opening and left and right lateral excursion are checked and abnormalities noted. The muscles of mastication are palpated for tenderness.

The maxillary sinuses

In disease these may give rise to swellings, to redness and tenderness over the cheek and canine fossa, to nasal discharge, and to fistulae into the mouth, often through a tooth socket.

The lymph nodes

The operator stands behind the patient, who flexes his head forward to relax his neck muscles. Enlarged submental and submandibular nodes can be felt with the finger tips by placing these below the lower border of the mandible and rolling the nodes outwards. The upper deep cervical group can be found by identifying the anterior border of the sternomastoid muscles and rolling the skin and subcutaneous tissues between fingers and thumb. With practice tenderness, consistency and degrees of mobility will be recognised.

The lips

These are inspected for lesions such as fissuring at the angles of the mouth, or ulceration.

Intraoral examination

The mucous membranes

The cheeks, lips, palate and floor of the mouth are examined for colour, texture and presence of swelling or ulceration. Comparison of both sides by palpation is essential to discover any abnormality.

The tongue

Movements, both intrinsic and extrinsic, are tested, as limitation is an important clinical sign in inflammation and early neoplasia. The dorsum is best seen by protruding the tongue over a dental napkin with which it can be grasped, drawn forward and, with the aid of a mouth mirror, examined over its length for fissures, ulcers, etc.

The tonsils

These are seen by depressing the tongue with a spatula and asking the patient to say 'Ah'. A second spatula compresses the anterior pillar of the fauces to evert the tonsil from its bed. Further pressure will expose and open the crypts.

The pharynx

Again the tongue is depressed, the patient asked to say 'Ah'. In a good light a small warm mirror is passed over the dorsum of the tongue, past the uvula, and rotated to show the naso- and oro-pharynx.

The salivary glands

The examination of these is described in Chapter 16.

The periodontal tissues

The colour and texture of the gingivae are noted, and the standard of oral hygiene classified including charting the presence of plaque and calculus. Recession, pocketing, and hyperplasia of the gums is measured, and the mobility of the teeth assessed.

The teeth

These are charted for caries and fillings with a mirror and probe. Loose teeth, crowns, or fillings are noted as these may have to be removed before a general anaesthetic is administered.

Edentulous ridges

These are examined for the form of the ridge, retained roots and soft tissue or bony abnormalities. Dentures worn should be inspected *in situ.*

The occlusion

This is best analysed by taking study models and mounting them on an anatomical articulator. However, the occlusal function of natural teeth, bridges and dentures should be assessed at the same time as the teeth are charted.

Special lesion

This is the examination of the lesion for which the patient has sought treatment. It may have been included in the general examination mentioned above, but frequently there is a swelling, ulcer, fistula or other disease which requires special attention, the details of which are best recorded under one heading easily referred to throughout treatment.

It is important in examining such pathological entities to determine their site, size, shape, colour, the character of their margins and whether they are single or multiple. Tenderness, discharge and lymphatic involvement are also important. Swellings should be palpated to determine whether they are mobile or fixed to the skin or to the underlying tissues. They may be either fluctuant or solid. Solid swellings may be very hard (like bone) or firm (like contracted muscle), soft (like relaxed muscle) or very soft (like fat). Where a collection of fluid is suspected fluctuation is elicited by placing two fingers of one hand on each side of the swelling and pressing centrally with a finger of the other hand. Where the lesion is fluid a thrill will be felt. This must be elicited in two directions at right angles as muscle fluctuates in the longitudinal but not the transverse plane. All pulsatile swellings must be checked to establish whether the pulsation is true or transmitted from an underlying artery.

Special investigation

The history taken, and the examination of the patient having been completed, the surgeon then considers his findings and makes a differential or provisional diagnosis. In this he wishes to establish the disease process and relate it to the tissue involved. It is a useful exercise for the inexperienced to consider in turn the chief pathological categories (Table 1.1) rejecting those that do not fit the facts ascertained. The tissues in the area may then be reviewed and an attempt

Table 1.1   The surgical sieve. The consideration of possible pathological processes and the tissues involved may be considered as a 'surgical sieve' into one of the holes of which the diagnosis may fit.

Pathological categories		Tissue involved									
		Epithelium	Connective tissue	Fat	Muscle	Bone	Blood vessels	Lymphatics	Nerves	Dental tissues	Salivary gland
Hereditary											
Developmental											
Traumatic											
Inflammatory	(acute)											
	(chronic)											
Cystic											
Neoplastic (benign)											
Neoplastic (malignant)											
Degenerative											
Medical											
Endocrine											

made to identify those from which the lesion could arise. In this way a sensible argument may be sustained to support one or more possible or differential diagnoses. To differentiate between these or to confirm a clinical finding special investigations may be necessary. These are not indicated for every patient; indeed, their cost and the delay involved in completing them make it necessary to limit their use. Such investigations are an aid to diagnosis and may also be required for treatment planning. It is convenient to divide the more usual procedures into the four main categories shown in Table 1.2.

Table 1.2   Special investigations commonly used in oral surgery.

Local dental investigations

A Performed in the surgery
  (1) Percussion of teeth for apical tenderness
  (2) Vitality tests on teeth
      (a) Thermal
      (b) Electrical
  (3) Radiography
  (4) Diagnostic injections of local anaesthetic solutions in facial pain
  (5) Study models for studying the occlusion
  (6) Photography as a comparative record

B Requiring special facilities
  (1) Bacteriological investigations including sensitivity tests
  (2) Aspiration of cystic cavities
  (3) Biopsy of tissue

General investigations

A Performed in the surgery
  (1) Temperature of body
  (2) Pulse rate
  (3) Blood pressure
  (4) Respiration rate

B Requiring special facilities
  (1) Urinalysis
      Physical examination for colour, specific gravity
      Chemical, tests for sugar, acetone, albumen, chlorides, blood
      Microscopic, examination for cells, bacteria, blood
      Bacteriological culture
  (2) Blood investigations
      Haemoglobin estimation
      Red cell, white cell and platelet count
      Bleeding and clotting mechanisms
      Grouping and cross matching for transfusion
      Blood chemistry and electrolytes – calcium, inorganic phosphorus, alkaline
          phosphatase, serum potassium, chloride, albumen, globulin, urea, glucose
          (see appendix)
      Serology
  (3) Chest radiographs
  (4) Electrocardiograph
  (5) Tests for allergy

Though the oral surgeon may not complete those tests requiring laboratory facilities, yet he must be quite clear about how the necessary specimens are collected and, even more important, understand the clinical significance of the results. These have been dealt with extensively in other works and the methods of collection of certain specimens are described later in this text in the appropriate chapter.

Diagnosis

When the special investigations have been completed the surgeon should be able to make a final diagnosis and it is important that this be clearly stated in the notes. Diagnosis is not a matter of intuition but is a 'computer' exercise in which all the information is sorted and analysed in the surgeon's mind. Sometimes it is impossible to reach a decision because of lack of information or knowledge, in which case the surgeon will need to consult textbooks or papers and will be wise to seek the opinion of a colleague.

Treatment planning

Only when the diagnosis is established can a satisfactory treatment plan be made. This should be divided into pre-operative, operative and post-operative care, each of which should be planned in a logical sequence, constantly bearing in mind that the ultimate aim is to cure the patient with the least risk and minimal inconvenience to him.

Further reading

Hill, G.L. & Farndon, J.R. (1994) *Guide for House Surgeons and Interns in the Surgical Unit*. Butterworth-Heinemann, Oxford.
Munro, J. & Edwards, C.R.W. (eds) (1995) *Macleod's Clinical Examination*, 9th edn. Churchill Livingstone, Edinburgh.

Chapter 2
General Patient Management

- Surgical patients
- In-patient care
- Intensive care
- Out-patient care
- Follow up

Surgical patients

The management of surgical patients can be considered under three headings: pre-operative, operative and post-operative; these should form a programme planned to meet the patient's therapeutic need. This chapter is concerned with the pre- and post-operative care, excluding the medically compromised patients, who are the subject of Chapter 3.

Once the operation has been planned it must be decided whether the patient requires admission to hospital, can be treated on a day-case basis or as an out-patient. The in-patient routine ensures a regular, ordered life with maximum rest. Much of the responsibility for the provision of care is entrusted to the nursing staff. Smoking is controlled and lights are turned out at 10.30 PM. Meals, although light and small in quantity, occur frequently at set intervals. This isolation from outside irritations provides an environment which, with the best will in the world, can seldom be achieved at home. Day-stay facilities where the patient is admitted in the morning to return home post-operatively, some hours after recovery, are becoming increasingly popular. The advantages are post-operative supervision by nursing staff during the period when complications related to surgery or anaesthesia may occur, whilst allowing the patient to return home at night. However the home circumstances must be such that the patient can be adequately looked after by relatives. The patient must be within reasonable distance of help postoperatively, should unexpected complications occur. In oral surgery the majority of out-patients are treated using local anaesthesia, sometimes in conjunction with sedation techniques. In-patients usually have endotracheal general anaesthesia of a longer duration than should be administered on a day-stay basis.

The indications for admitting patients to hospital are surgical, medical and social.

Surgical

The diagnosis is in doubt and further investigations are needed, the risk of complications such as haemorrhage or fracture of the jaw exists, multiple operations are proposed, or major surgery is being undertaken. In the last respect size alone is no criterion of the importance of the condition.

Medical

The patient requires collateral treatment by a physician, needs special therapy or skilled nursing care.

Social

The patient's home conditions are poor, he is living alone, lives far away or he is anxious to be treated as an in-patient.

In-patient care demands a wider application of the general principles which underlie the management of surgical patients. It is therefore considered first, though no important difference is implied between the needs of in- and out-patients.

In-patient care

The date of admission to hospital can be arranged at the time of consultation and waiting lists thereby avoided. Where a waiting list is used it is important to give adequate warning that a bed is available and also to recognise certain surgical priorities such as the following.

Emergency

Conditions requiring instant admission such as acute infections or traumatic injuries.

Urgent

Conditions which can progress to emergencies if treatment is long delayed, for example subacute infections, and neoplasms.

Routine

Those of no urgency who may take their turn in chronological order.

A patient who is fit and only requires routine surgery is normally admitted the day before the operation. Where special preparation is needed, such as blood investigation, the fitting of splints or consultation with other specialists, the time of admission must be calculated to allow for these procedures to take place first.

Within a few hours of admission the patient should be visited by the surgeon and findings made at the out-patient examination reviewed and revised if necessary. The pulse, temperature, blood pressure, haemoglobin estimation and urinalysis are recorded. The mouth must be carefully examined and the teeth assessed to enable those beyond conservation to be extracted under the same anaesthetic. Insecure dressings should be replaced to prevent their being dislodged into a socket or wound. Before a general anaesthetic loose or crowned teeth are noted and the anaesthetist warned. Where extensive haemorrhage is anticipated blood is taken for grouping and cross matching, and the necessary amount for replacement is ordered. Where grouping is done only as a precautionary measure the serum may be kept for cross matching if required but no blood ordered. The nature of the operation and likely complications should be explained to the patient and informed consent obtained in writing for both the anaesthetic and the operation.

It is the role of the oral surgeon not only to carry out the local treatment but also to supervise the day-to-day care.

Relations with the nursing staff

The dental surgeon must understand the routine of the wards and the way his patients are nursed. Though it is essential to make daily visits to assess progress and give treatment, these must be arranged to avoid awkward times when the wards are normally closed. The nursing staff spend much time with the patient and have opportunities to hear complaints and observe minor changes which the surgeon may overlook. Their comments can therefore be of great help and they should be consulted about progress daily.

Informed consent

Before any procedure is undertaken the patient's informed consent must be obtained. The proposed operation or investigation should be explained in simple language which can be understood by the lay person. The commoner complications must be mentioned without causing undue distress. Where a general anaesthetic or sedation is proposed the consent should be in writing. For those under sixteen years of age, it must be given by their parent or guardian.

Major points on informed consent:

- For any surgical procedure on children under 16
- For all patients undergoing general anaesthesia or sedation
- Requires careful explanation by staff who fully understand the procedure
- Full warnings of recognised complications must be noted
- Nervous patients may have little recall of information given

Diet

A knowledge of the principles of nutrition is essential to understand the dietetic problems of the patient, and the following summary is presented with this in mind. The diet can be broadly divided into its fluid and solid content.

Fluid intake and output

The water intake is approximately the sum of the weight, expressed in grammes, of fluid and of solid food ingested, because solid food when digested and metabolised yields three-fifths its own weight as water. The water intake should be about 2500 ml daily, half of which is taken as drinks.

Water is excreted as exhaled air, 400 ml, evaporation including sweat 500–1000 ml, urine 1200 ml, and faeces 200 ml. Water lost by exhalation and evaporation is used for heat regulation and the quantity lost varies widely according to the circumstances. Insufficient fluid intake shows as a decrease in urine output. The absolute daily minimum of urine is the 600 ml required to carry the 50 g of urinary solids excreted daily; below this toxic metabolites are returned to the blood. At this concentration the specific gravity is raised from 1.015 to 1.030. All patients who have difficulty in feeding because of acute trismus or mouth injuries should have a fluid balance chart. This shows on the credit side all fluid taken in 24 hours including metabolic water, and on the debit side the urine passed plus an estimate for water lost by evaporation which may be very high in febrile states. For all practical purposes the urine output is a measure of the water balance.

In the adult the daily output should be at least 1000–1500 ml. This simple but accurate criterion is satisfactory unless cardiovascular or renal disease is present, when over-enthusiastic pressing of fluids beyond the power of the kidney to excrete may result in waterlogging of the tissues. Fluids may be administered by several routes, of which only the oral and intravenous are much used. The safest, most convenient and effective way of giving fluids is by mouth if not contraindicated and should be preferred to all others. Up to three litres of water, flavoured attractively, can be taken each day. Where the intraoral route cannot be used fluids may be given intravenously.

Solid food

A balanced diet includes carbohydrates, fats, proteins, vitamins and mineral salts.

Fats, the highest calorie provider, are not easily digested by the sick and their intake may have to be markedly reduced. They are, however, important as a vehicle for the fat-soluble vitamins A, D, E and K. In starvation the body's fat reserves may be mobilised, but a certain minimum daily quantity of carbohydrate is needed for their physiological use and to prevent ketosis. Only 100 g of glycogen is stored in the liver, which is less than a one-day requirement. Protein is essential for the repair of tissues, and for maintaining the circulation.

A deficiency may occur after extensive haemorrhage or burns and may increase the susceptibility to shock, impede the healing of wounds, impair circulatory efficiency, and lower resistance to infection. Patients in bed undergo protein wastage which is best prevented by a high carbohydrate and protein diet. Vitamins and mineral salts are essential and are supplied therapeutically, if deficient.

Food must be attractively prepared, and even if sieved or in fluid form it should not lose its identity. Each meal should bear some resemblance to its usual form; most foods can be easily liquidised and baby foods though expensive are useful in this respect.

Special dietary requirements must be discussed with the dietitian and the ward sister. The total calories, the amount of water, protein and vitamins, together with proprietary preparations and the number and the kind of supplementary feeds, must be specified. The rule 'a little and often' will help to avoid indigestion, and to ensure an adequate intake particularly when the jaws are wired together. Supplementary feeds should be considered so that the daily routine includes early morning tea, breakfast, 'elevenses', lunch, tea, dinner, supper and nightcap.

Certain patients may have to be fed through a nasogastric (Ryle's) tube. This is a small-bore plastic tube passed through the nose so that about 5 cm lies in the stomach. The normal length of tube from the nose is 50 cm; any excess interferes with gastric peristalsis and may cause anorexia and nausea. Its presence in the stomach is confirmed by radiographs if possible or by aspirating gastric contents up the tube before feeding is started. Feeding may be continued in this way indefinitely if, every two or three days, the tube is brought out, cleaned and replaced through the other nostril. Feed is pumped from a calibrated dispenser at a controlled rate to ensure that it is tolerated. This is initiated at 5 ml/hour and gradually increased to full strength over 24 to 48 hours. Before disconnecting the syringe the nasogastric tube must be clamped off. All patients on special diets should be weighed weekly as a check on their progress.

Pre-operative diet

Patients for operation under local anaesthesia may take their normal meals. If the patient has missed a meal he should be given a glucose drink before the injection is given. Where a general anaesthetic is to be administered a light meal, chiefly of protein and carbohydrate, is advised the night before. On the day of operation those on the morning list are starved, but those for the afternoon list may be given a small breakfast of tea and toast. No food must be taken for 4 hours nor clear fluids for 2 hours before operation.

Post-operative diet

Each patient must be considered individually, but feeding should be started as soon as possible to avoid nausea. Many can manage the ordinary fare provided, but others, because of tenderness or trismus, require specially prepared food. Where necessary, before discharge home the patient should receive dietary advice.

Excretion

Micturition

This reflex act occurs when the pressure in the bladder rises sufficiently to cause the sphincter to relax and the detrusor muscle to contract. The ability to delay micturition is the inhibition of the normal reflex response to distension. In patients with head injuries the apparently insane desire to get out of bed is often for the purpose of emptying the bladder or bowel, as the wish to go to the right place is strongly imbued and may persist despite gross craniocerebral disturbance. Retention can be organic, as in men suffering from prostatic enlargement, or a functional disorder. It may occur after general anaesthesia but should cause no undue anxiety up to 24 hours unless the bladder becomes distended or symptoms of overflow occur. Micturition can be encouraged by getting the patient up but if this fails catheterisation may be necessary.

Sweat

Sweat contains 0.5 per cent of solids, chiefly sodium chloride. In fever or in hot weather sweating may be greatly increased and as much as 10 g of sodium chloride can be lost in an hour, which must be replaced in the diet.

Defaecation

The bowels should be regularly opened and the fact noted but too much attention can be paid to irregularity. In constipation one must first decide whether the cause is organic or functional. Organic is due to partial obstruction of the lumen, often by a tumour. Functional may be due to defective movements of the colonic musculature, or a deficiency in bulk of faeces due to feeding with fluid diets. It may arise in hospital as a result of a sudden change in routine and of diet.

It is treated either by feeding fruit, vegetables and wholemeal cereals or by giving laxatives. It is stressed that wherever there is doubt as to the cause a general surgeon's opinion should be sought.

Sleep

Sleep is distinguished from other unconscious states by the ease with which the sleeper may be roused. Disturbed sleep may be due to pain, to external stimuli, to worry or to change of habit. It is important to recognise the cause before considering treatment. Where this is pain, hypnotics must not be given until its source has been investigated, removed if possible, or analgesics prescribed. If these are effective the patient should sleep naturally. External stimuli should be reduced by keeping the wards dark at night, and by providing side wards for night admissions and for the noisy or restless patients. Worry or change of habit, particularly dozing by day, can lead to insomnia in the convalescent or fit adult. Hypnotic drugs may be prescribed, but only if really necessary for they are habit-forming.

Hygiene

General and oral hygiene is the responsibility of the ward sister, but mouth hygiene is supervised by the dental surgeon. On admission the patient should be given a dental prophylaxis and instructed in oral hygiene.

In the badly injured, the elderly and in those recently operated upon, a modified technique is necessary either to avoid causing pain or because they need assistance. No cleansing of the mouth is advised for the first 24 hours after operation and may indeed do harm by starting haemorrhage. Thereafter, mucous membranes and teeth may be cleansed with a soft tooth-brush or foam pads attached to orange sticks, and the mouth irrigated with 0.2 per cent aqueous chlorhexidine after every meal. Intraoral sutures also require care as they tend to trap food over the wound. Clinging debris should be removed by swabbing with cotton wool each day. A hypertonic saline mouth bath may be used as hot as the individual can bear without scalding and allowed to lie over the wound until cool, but unlike the mouth-washes used pre-operatively, no violent flushing is advised. Mouth-brushing is started on normal teeth and gingivae as soon as possible and the patient encouraged at an early stage to carry out his own oral hygiene. This not only occupies his time usefully, but the techniques may be supervised before discharge, ensuring satisfactory home care.

Arch bars

Arch bars may be cleaned with a toothbrush and paste and chlorhexidine mouthwash can be employed with obturators.

Where gutta-percha moulds are used to hold skin grafts in position the mouth is cleansed using only the blandest mouthwashes. After the first ten days (by which time the graft should have taken) a syringe may be introduced between the graft and the mould to clean the dead space gently but thoroughly.

Premedication and sedation

See Chapter 5.

Post-operative care

On arriving in the recovery room after an operation the patient is immediately put into bed and laid on his side with a pillow behind his shoulders in the position of sleep in such a way that drainage may take place from his mouth. His arms are kept folded over his chest. Under no circumstances should the arms be elevated above his head for fear of damage to the brachial plexus.

During the uneasy period before complete consciousness is regained, and especially where the jaws are wired together, a nurse must sit with the patient to watch the airway, suck out the mouth and oro-pharynx, ensure that he does himself no injury by pulling at sutures or splints or, as can happen, falls out of bed. She also watches for vomiting and haemorrhage, and records the pulse, blood pressure, respirations and level of consciousness.

Post-operative medication

Analgesics should be given to reduce post-operative pain. Hypnotics should not be prescribed for semi-conscious patients where the jaws are wired together (see Chapter 5).

Post-operative complications

These can include fever, vomiting, conjunctivitis, sore throat, pharyngitis and pulmonary conditions.

Fever

Raised temperature is a natural reaction to infection but a slight fever is common for two to three days after an operation where a haematoma or necrotic material is present. A large haematoma may keep the temperature up for a week. After a general anaesthetic a chest complaint as a cause of fever must be considered and any sputum sent for culture. More rarely a temporary upset of heat regulation does occur after an anaesthetic or a head injury.

The primary treatment must be that of the underlying cause whether local or general. The symptomatic treatment includes confinement to bed, liberal administration of fluids and a high carbohydrate diet which has been found to prevent the breakdown of body proteins. At temperatures of 39.4°C and over, the body may be sponged down with tepid water at 27°C which cools the patient and refreshes him.

Vomiting

This does occur following operation, usually due to the anaesthetic or swallowed blood, though the nervous disposition of the patient is a factor. Persistent vomiting for more than eight hours is part of a vicious circle characterised by an upset of the acid base equilibrium, in which the alkali reserve is reduced with increased urinary acidity and ketonuria. For the treatment of this the anaesthetist should be consulted. It can however often be avoided by energetic treatment earlier. This consists of giving milk or alkaline drinks with glucose, which should be sipped very slowly but frequently. An antiemetic may be prescribed (Chapter 5).

Conjunctivitis

Conjunctivitis can be caused by anaesthetic vapours, blood, antiseptics or towels entering the eye, or by the eye being open and drying up during the operation. This can be prevented by keeping the eyes closed with eyepads, but should contamination occur the eye can be gently irrigated with normal saline. Chloramphenicol eye-drops will afford relief.

Sore throat or pharyngitis

This is usually caused by trauma from the endotracheal tube, excoriation from a dry pack or desiccation following use of atropine. It may be treated with gargles and inhalations (Chapter 5).

Pulmonary complications

Routine post-operative breathing exercises will reduce the incidence of pulmonary complications but it must be borne in mind that these may occur. They may range from a minor inflammation of the trachea or bronchi to pulmonary collapse or post-operative pneumonia. Where they are suspected a chest radiograph should be taken and the anaesthetist immediately informed. Their general management will include the use of antibiotics, physiotherapy, humidified oxygen, sedatives and mucolytic drugs. Frequent hot drinks help to relieve spasm and loosen secretions.

Progress

Routine monitoring of in-patients should include:

- Vital signs:
  - temperature, pulse, blood pressure
- Fluid balance chart
- Bloods:
  - full blood count, haemoglobin, electrolytes
- Bowel habit
- Dietary intake
- Drug requirements:
  - analgesics, antibiotics, normal medications

The patient should be visited daily by the surgeon, who should first ask the patient how he feels and about his day-to-day care, diet and oral hygiene. This is followed by a careful examination of the operation site, a check of the temperature chart, drug sheet, etc., and questions to the nursing staff where necessary. The response to treatment is assessed and should be recorded in the notes, together with any changes to be made in the treatment. Before discharge the patient's final condition should be summarised. The importance of these records cannot be overstressed as it is difficult to compare progress over a long period without them.

Discharge

When the patient is fit for discharge home the patient or the relatives must be informed of the regime and treatment to be followed and when to attend for review. Sick benefit notes must be completed and adequate transport, if necessary, arranged both to the patient's home and for his return for review.

The patient's doctor and dental surgeon should receive notification that the patient is being discharged, including an outline of the operative procedures and condition on discharge. In this way, if called in an emergency, they are informed of all that has gone before, and they are able to prescribe for any drugs or dressings required at home.

Intensive care

Not all patients will follow the above routine; some will be admitted shocked, unconscious or both. Some will require special management after operation and the condition of others may deteriorate whilst they are on the ward. In the modern hospital the critically ill patients are treated in an intensive care unit by specialised staff.

The management of respiration may require intubation or tracheostomy and, on occasion, the use of a mechanical ventilator. Such care is entirely within the realm of a specialist anaesthetist. Fluids and feeding for these patients is often given intravenously. All prolonged intravenous infusion requires the most careful continual monitoring as it is all too easy to upset the delicately balanced homeostasis.

Intravenous fluids

The solution must be sterile and is contained in a bottle or bag into which a polythene tube is inserted. All air should be removed from the tube by running the fluid through it with the stop clamp open. A suitable vein, not too superficial nor near a joint, is chosen and a tourniquet is placed above the selected point. An indwelling plastic cannula is inserted over a needle, which is then withdrawn, and the giving set attached. The cannula is secured in place and the flow adjusted according to the patient's needs. Usually this is about 1 litre over 8 hours.

The fluids that may be given in this way are whole blood, plasma and saline, dextrose or fat solutions. The decision as to which fluid to use will depend on the clinical needs of the patient. Blood may be given as a replacement following loss from trauma or surgery and saline or dextrose solutions during long operations and the immediate recovery period; where the use of intravenous fluids goes beyond this short term, monitoring is performed using a central venous pressure line and by taking blood samples and estimating blood sugar and electrolytes. Where feeding using fat solutions is necessary urinary urea estimation and body weight will indicate the nitrogen to be replaced and the calories required.

Out-patient care

All the principles of management of in-patient care, particularly those relating to diet, hygiene and progress, are applicable with modification to out-patients. The salient points with regard to outpatients are summarised here.

Day cases

Where out-patients are having minor operations under endotracheal anaesthesia they may be operated during the morning but kept in a suitably equipped recovery room or ward under adequate professional and nursing supervision. As it is usual for these patients to stay on the premises all day and be discharged home in the evening they are known as 'day cases' although otherwise their general care is the same as that of other out-patients. However they must be adequately assessed and height/weight criteria may be applicable before they are accepted for out-patient anaesthesia. Suitable transport must be available and they will require rest and care on their return home. Careful enquiry should be made as to the patient's home circumstances to ensure that adequate support can be provided.

Finally both the anaesthetist and the surgeon should be able and experienced in their fields so that the patient is not exposed to risk due to lack of skill or judgement.

Pre-assessment clinics

Nurse-run pre-assessment clinics (PAC) are often used to improve day-case services. The patient attends some weeks before surgery and the details of the patient's fitness to undergo surgery are confirmed. The consent is checked and the patient encouraged to ask questions about the procedure in order to allay fears. The date of the surgery is confirmed to minimise the chance of non-attendance.

Pre-operative instructions for out-patients

The nature of the operation must be explained and the patient's permission obtained in writing for both general anaesthetic and surgery. Out-patients should be told to come accompanied and whether it will be safe to take alcohol, drive a car or bicycle, or operate machinery (including cooking). Instructions should be given about diet before a local anaesthetic – something light and easily digested. Where a general anaesthetic is to be administered they are instructed to come accompanied, to wear no restrictive clothing and to fast from food or drink for at least 4 hours before operation; in this respect children require particular supervision. Patients having sedation should be given similar instructions to those having a general anaesthetic. Of particular importance is the advice that the patient must not drive a motor vehicle or operate machinery until the following day. Before entering the surgery they are asked to remove their dentures, contact lenses and earrings, and to empty bowel and bladder.

Pre-operative dental treatment

Pre-operative prophylaxis and instruction in oral hygiene is given to those about to undergo a dental operation. Many patients fail to appreciate the importance of this measure, All doubtful teeth should be assessed and insecure dressings replaced so that those beyond conservation can be extracted under the same anaesthetic. Before a general anaesthetic very loose teeth should be noted and the anaesthetist warned.

Pre- and post-medication

This is discussed in Chapter 5.

Post-operative care

Before dismissing the patient, a reasonable time should be allowed for recovery. This applies equally to those treated under local or general anaesthesia, and particularly to day case patients.

Adequate instructions should be given for home treatment. If possible these should be stated in the presence of a relative or written, as the patient may not be sufficiently alert after the surgical ordeal to remember details. These should include diet, oral hygiene, analgesics and the rest period required before return to work. The date and time of the next appointment must also be clearly stated, together with the action to be taken should a post-operative emergency, such as haemorrhage, arise (Table 2.1).

The operator *must be easily available* to the patient to deal with any surgical complications which may arise. Where a general anaesthetic has been given, the general medical practitioner should be informed.

Follow-up

It is the duty of the surgeon to assume responsibility for the patient's after-care until all possibility of post-operative complications is past. Although it is often tedious, long-term follow-up should be carried out personally, as through it much may be learned which will benefit both the surgeon and his patients.

Table 2.1 Specimen of post-operative instructions to patient.

To prevent bleeding:
   AVOID mouthwashing for 24 hours
               hot drinks, hot food and alcohol
               exercise or effort

If bleeding occurs:
   Apply pressure by biting on to a clean rolled handkerchief
   Rest sitting in an upright position
   If bleeding is not controlled by these measures contact us by telephone by day on
      xxxx–xxxx, by night on xxxx–xxxx.

If in pain:
   Take two paracetamol tablets
   If pain is persistent or severe contact the dental surgery

After 24 hours:
   Mix one teaspoonful of salt in a tumbler of hot water
   Take a mouthful and tilt head so that the water lies over the extraction site.
   Hold water over area, spit it out and repeat until the tumbler is empty

Operation . . . .
Anaesthetic . . . .

Before final discharge, the surgeon should refer back through the notes and establish that not only have the operations been successful, but that the patient has been relieved of his original complaint and that any subsequent complications incurred during treatment have been cured.

Further reading

Campbell, D. & Spence, A.A. (1997) *Norris and Campbell's Anaesthetics, Resuscitation, and Intensive Care.* Churchill Livingstone, New York.
Ganong, W.F. (1999) *Review of Medical Physiology*, 19th edn. Prentice Hall International.

Chapter 3
Problems Related to Certain Systemic Conditions

- Physiological conditions
- Endocrine diseases
- Allergy
- Cardiovascular disorders
- Ventricular shunts and prosthetic joints
- Disorders of the blood
- Respiratory disorders
- Infectious diseases
- Epilepsy
- Systemic diseases of bone
- Depressive illness

Patients referred for oral surgery may often be suffering from systemic diseases or undergoing treatment with drugs, either of which may complicate the operation, including the choice and administration of an anaesthetic. Where surgical procedures cause an exacerbation of the medical condition it is the physician who will treat it, not the oral surgeon. Nothing is more calculated to annoy a general medical practitioner than to be called unexpectedly to advise one of his chronically ill patients who has undergone a surgical operation about which he has not been informed.

A full medical history is therefore essential and should be rechecked periodically if the patient attends for a prolonged period. Whenever a patient is under treatment by a physician the latter must be informed of the proposed operation and his co-operation sought with the pre- and post-operative care, particularly with regard to the special precautions necessary for the disease. No alteration should be made to the drug regime without such prior consultation. Advances in drug therapy occur rapidly and where a patient is on medication with which the oral surgeon is not familiar reference should be made to the British National Formulary.

The more important conditions commonly met in practice will now be discussed.

Physiological conditions

Menstruation

This is not a contraindication to surgery except that patients are often depressed physically and mentally, and this time is best avoided. It has been stated that haemorrhage after extractions is prolonged, but no increase in the bleeding or clotting time of clinical significance has been demonstrated.

Pregnancy

In general, women in pregnancy undergo operations and anaesthesia well, if not better than at other times. The physical or psychological trauma of extraction does not endanger the foetus though it may be blamed for so doing. A local anaesthetic with adrenalin is satisfactory as the hormonal mechanism shields the uterus from smooth muscle activators. In general anaesthesia the greatest danger to the foetus is anoxia, which, even if slight, may have serious, even fatal, results at any time. This is most likely to occur later in pregnancy, especially in the last three months, because the size of the uterus reduces the vital capacity of the mother's lungs, and because the oxygen supply to the human foetus in a normal pregnancy falls slowly to the thirty sixth week and rapidly thereafter. If general anaesthesia during pregnancy is unavoidable the procedure should be undertaken in an in-patient facility with all care taken to avoid anoxia.

The optimum time for operation is the second trimester, i.e. fourth, fifth and sixth months of pregnancy because at that time the danger to the foetus is least. Spontaneous abortion occurs most frequently in the first trimester and the foetus is more at risk from teratogenic drugs, thus care should be taken when prescribing during this time. The last trimester of pregnancy should be avoided in view of the possibility of precipitating premature labour. Certain patients give a history of habitual abortion at other times, and for these surgery should not be undertaken at that particular time.

Many expectant mothers suffer from anaemia, and as this may increase the danger of anoxia to the foetus, the haemoglobin level should be ascertained before any operation is commenced.

Endocrine diseases

Hyperthyroidism

In hyperthyroidism either oral surgery or the injection of local anaesthetic containing adrenalin may precipitate a thyroid crisis. For these reasons surgery must be delayed until the physician is satisfied that the patient is adequately prepared. A general anaesthetic may be preferable to local anaesthesia as it is less upsetting psychologically.

Adrenal corticosteroids

The adrenal cortex produces hormones which are of importance to the surgeon since among their functions they affect the balance of electrolytes, depress the inflammatory response and play a large part in the body's reaction to stress. Their secretion is stimulated by the adrenocorticotrophic hormone (ACTH), produced by the anterior lobe of the pituitary. When the amount of adreno-cortical hormone in the circulation reaches the necessary level, production of ACTH is inhibited.

Corticosteroids or their synthetic equivalents are used in medicine for replacement therapy of insufficiency which may be chronic primary as in Addison's disease, or chronic secondary as in hypopituitarism. They are also used in the treatment of a wide variety of medical conditions including asthma and the collagen diseases. Where the blood level of the adrenocortical steroids is kept high for therapeutic purposes the adrenal cortex atrophies and causes an iatrogenic insufficiency. Any sudden demand under conditions of stress cannot be met, with the result that an acute adrenal insufficiency (Addisonian crisis) may occur with all the signs and symptoms of shock. Depression of function may continue for 2 years after their therapeutic use has stopped and those who require a general anaesthetic or surgery must have adequate premedication with steroids. At present this is 100 mg hydrocortisone sodium succinate given IM or IV. In addition the patient's blood pressure should be monitored at intervals during the procedure and for a period afterwards. Evidence is emerging that patients on long term steroids are less at risk of an Addisonian crisis than previously thought and in future this protocol may be revised in the light of further research. Should a crisis supervene 200 mg should be injected at once intravenously or intramuscularly together with 1 ml of 1:1000 adrenalin given subcutaneously. An intravenous transfusion should be started of 0.9 per cent (154 m.mols/l) saline, containing a second 100 mg of the hydrocortisone sodium succinate. This therapy may be repeated.

Diabetes

Diabetes mellitus is a disease characterised by a rise in blood sugar, excretion of sugar and acetone in the urine, and an increased susceptibility to infection. Emotional stress or infection may increase the severity of the disease. Broadly the patients may be considered in two groups. The elderly group, often overweight, develop diabetes later in life. They are non-insulin-dependent diabetics and are treated where necessary with oral hypoglycaemic agents. The second group are insulin-dependent diabetics. Their management is more complex and requires the administration of insulin. In uncontrolled diabetes, hyperglycaemic coma may occur, but this is of slow onset and the patient is so obviously ill beforehand that it is unlikely to present as an emergency in the dental surgery.

However, hypoglycaemia (insulin shock) can occur with alarming suddenness in patients on insulin who have taken insufficient carbohydrate. Weakness, hunger, pallor, a rapid pulse and profuse sweating herald its onset, which if severe is followed by confusion and loss of consciousness. Treatment is to give sugar by mouth or 1 mg glucagon intramuscularly. The patient must be observed to ensure that treatment is adequate.

Where a diabetic is to have an operation under local anaesthesia he should take his normal diet and insulin at the usual time and the operation should be commenced about one hour after. It is not necessary to use adrenalin-free local anaesthetic solutions, but the operation must not be unduly prolonged, nor must meals or snacks on the patient's schedule be missed.

Those on insulin who have an acute infection or need a general anaes-thetic should undoubtedly be admitted to hospital, where the advice of a physi-cian may be sought. When a general anaesthetic is to be given the physician will manage the case according to the following broad principles. Those on long-acting insulin are changed to the soluble form and rebalanced. All but the most severe diabetics will then receive their normal insulin and carbohy-drate till midnight on the day before operation. Next morning they should be operated first and are given only a saline infusion during the operation, after which a blood sugar estimation is immediately performed before administering the necessary insulin and glucose by infusion. Post-operatively, careful moni-toring of the patient and urine testing is continued till the normal balance is resumed.

For severe diabetics or where a long operation is involved, more complicated management may be required involving a glucose, potassium and insulin infusion (GKI).

The surgeon must take measures to control infection at the site of operation by careful oral prophylaxis; dentures are provided as quickly as possible so that the patient can resume his normal diet.

Allergy

Anaphylaxis

See Chapter 4.

Angioedema

Angioedema is a disease in which there is widespread oedema due to increased vascular permeability as a result of an allergic reaction. Two forms exist; one is hereditary and is an apparently exaggerated response to minor trauma and is characteristically shared by other members of the family. The disease is due to a lack of C1 esterase inhibitor and a consequent initiation of the complement cascade. Administration of fresh frozen plasma (FFP) prior to surgery provides sufficient inhibitor to prevent the problem. In the event of a spontaneous angioedamatous attack the patient is treated with steroids.

The non-hereditary variety is a kind of urticaria in which there is an allergic response not only to food and drugs, but also to emotional situations. Trauma seldom produces serious complications but the use of allergenic substances may do so. Should an acute reaction occur it should be treated as for anaphylactic shock described in Chapter 4.

Cardiovascular disorders

There are many heart conditions but the dental surgeon is concerned firstly with those which affect the efficiency of the heart as a pump, and secondly those where the valvular endocardium is damaged and susceptible to infection.

Hypertension

Hypertensive patients can trouble the dental surgeon in two ways. First, the raised blood pressure may be a cause of post-operative bleeding as it may prevent the normal vascular and platelet mechanism from arresting haemorrhage effectively. Second, those under treatment with anti-hypertensive drugs can be more susceptible to the hypotensive effects of general anaesthetics, making it necessary to inform the anaesthetist of their use.

Coronary artery disease

Disease of the coronary vessels, because it causes ischaemia of the heart muscle, affects the efficiency of the heart as a pump. Where partial occlusion of the vessels is present severe pain of short duration, called angina of effort, occurs during physical or emotional stress because the demand for blood by the myocardium outstrips the possible supply. Treatment includes the use of vasodilators when pain is experienced. Details of the frequency of need for these tablets will give an indication of the severity of the disease. Where use of the drug is frequent, or increasing in frequency, advice should be sought from the patient's physician. Complete occlusion of a coronary artery is known as a coronary thrombosis, when the patient has acute pain of long duration, resulting in a myocardial infarction (MI), which may be fatal.

Patients suffering from coronary disease should be treated in conjunction with a physician and should be admitted when a general anaesthetic is required.

Some may be on treatment with anticoagulants and obviously require special preparation (see later). Those operated under local anaesthesia may require premedication to allay anxiety, and to be kept in the supine position to reduce strain on the heart. In unstable angina the use of a local anaesthetic solution containing octapressin is indicated, otherwise lignocaine and adrenaline may be used; however the quantity of any local anaesthetic solution should always be strictly monitored and the amount limited to half the safe levels in a normal patient of the same age. Those using glyceryl trinitrate tablets or sublingual spray may be asked to use them before the operation starts – the vasodilator effect lasts about half an hour.

Should an anginal attack occur, the patient is laid down and a sublingual glyceryl trinitrate spray should be administered. Oxygen is administered at 6 litres/minute. Where the severity of the attack is marked by cyanosis, cold sweat and dyspnoea suggesting a coronary thrombosis the patient is laid down, given oxygen, and morphine sulphate 20 mg subcutaneously to ease the pain. The patient should be referred to hospital and not sent directly home.

Cardiac failure

The symptoms of heart failure are a reduced exercise tolerance, cyanosis, dyspnoea and oedema of the lower extremities. The patient in early failure may not present with these but leads an apparently normal life. Although he has a loss of cardiac reserve this is apparent only when the extra demands made by physical exercise or hypoxia cannot be met.

Failure of the heart to act as an efficient pump occurs in many diseases including congenital heart disease, cardiac arrhythmias, hyperthyroidism, coronary heart disease, hypertension and rheumatic carditis. Patients suffering from these should not be operated on without a physician's advice as those in failure may be greatly improved by admission to hospital for bed rest and medical treatment. The anaesthetic of choice for these patients is a local anaesthetic. Premedication with a suitable anxiolytic drug should be considered if the patient is unduly concerned about the proposed operation.

Infective endocarditis

Antibiotic cover is required:

- In patients with heart valve lesions
- In patients with septal defects or patent ductus
- In patients with prosthetic heart valves
- In patients with a history of bacterial endocarditis

The endocardium of the heart valves may be damaged, as happens in certain congenital heart diseases, in rheumatic fever and Huntington's chorea or following cardiac surgery. The dental surgeon must realise that in these cases the heart may function completely satisfactorily as a pump, yet it may still be susceptible to infection from a bacteraemia at any time during the patient's life. Among infecting organisms *Streptococcus viridans* has repeatedly been shown to be released into the blood stream during tooth extraction or oral prophylaxis.

Protection may be required for those with a history of congenital heart disease or rheumatic fever, or who have had cardiac valvular surgery as advised by a cardiologist. Typically this may be one dose of 3 g amoxycillin orally one hour pre-operatively. For those who are allergic to penicillin oral clindamycin 600 mg is given one hour pre-operatively. For those having a general anaesthetic, 1 mg amoxycillin may be given by intravenous injection followed by 500 mg orally six hours later.

Special risk

Where there is a history of an episode of endocarditis or the patient has prosthetic replacement of a heart valve, 1 g amoxycillin and 1.5 mg/kg gentamicin are given intramuscularly to be followed by 500 mg oral amoxycillin six hours later. For this latter group who are allergic to penicillin, intravenous teicoplanin and gentamicin are given.

Ventricular shunts and prosthetic joints

Patients suffering from congenital hydrocephalus may have artificial valves inserted to relieve intracranial pressure. There is no evidence to suggest that these are at risk of infection when a bacteraemia occurs. There is an increase in the number of patients receiving prosthetic joint replacements of hip and knee. In the past these patients have received antibiotics prior to dental extraction; however there is no evidence to suggest that these prostheses are susceptible to infection from bacteraemias during dental treatment.

Disorders of the blood

Anaemia

The oral surgeon must satisfy himself that the patient is not clinically anaemic before operation, and where doubt exists a haemoglobin estimation and blood film examination must be performed. It should always be remembered that there are several different forms of anaemia and that it can be symptomatic of serious disease such as leukaemia, which requires investigation by a haematologist. In severe anaemia, operation is delayed until it has responded to treatment or in an emergency a blood transfusion has been arranged.

Sickle cell anaemia

This haemoglobinopathy is a hereditary disease found in individuals of African, Asian and Mediterranean origin. The abnormal haemoglobin (HbS) in lowered oxygen tension (such as may occur during a general anaesthetic) results in the red corpuscle becoming sickle-shaped, leading to an increased blood viscosity and capillary thrombosis. It can present either as true sickle cell anaemia or as sickle cell trait in which there is a variable proportion of affected haemoglobin, the remainder being normal.

All patients who may have inherited the disease and require a general anaesthetic should be tested for sickling (sickledex test). Positive patients require further investigation by a haematologist to differentiate those with the trait from those with sickle cell anaemia. Both groups are more safely treated under local anaesthesia, but where a general anaesthetic is necessary the patient should be referred to hospital for a specialist anaesthetic opinion.

Thalassaemias

These inherited diseases are seen in Mediterranean races in whom foetal haemoglobin continues to be produced after birth. The patients suffer from haemolytic anaemia and should be treated in hospital.

Leukaemias

All forms of leukaemia are a contraindication to any form of oral surgery without full investigation and advice from a haematologist, owing to the difficulty of controlling post-operative bleeding and infection. In such cases a conservative approach to dental care should be adopted until the leukaemia is in remission or the patient is free of the disease.

Haemorrhagic diseases

The natural arrest of haemorrhage is brought about in three ways, first by the contraction of the vessel walls, second by plugging of small deficiencies by platelets, and third by the clotting of the blood. Clinically, patients with haemorrhagic disease can be divided into those where bleeding is profuse at operation and continues – these have a prolonged bleeding time but clotting may be normal – and those where bleeding usually stops for a short period after operation but persistent haemorrhage occurs later owing to failure of the blood to clot – these may have a normal bleeding time, but an abnormality of coagulation.

Prolonged bleeding time

This is found where vascular damage prevents arrest by the contraction of the walls of cut vessels or in platelet abnormalities in which there is ineffective plugging of small deficiencies.

Disorders of blood vessels

These occur in anaphylactoid (allergic) purpura of Henoch and Schönlein, in symptomatic purpura as in scurvy, in severe infections such as scarlet fever, following the use of certain drugs, and in hereditary haemorrhagic telangiectasia.

Platelet abnormalities

These are of two kinds: thrombocytopenic purpuras where there is a low platelet count which may be primary as in idiopathic purpura or secondary to drugs or other blood diseases such as leukaemia; and thrombocythaemic purpura in which the platelet count is greatly raised, the condition being related to polycythaemia.

Abnormal coagulation

Table 3.1 shows the clotting mechanism. There are several theories, of which the waterfall concept is one. The extrinsic mechanism is activated by damaged tissue, whereas the intrinsic is activated by contact of blood with a surface other than blood cells or endothelium.

Coagulation defects are rare and may arise from a deficiency of any of the factors concerned in the mechanism. The most common disease due to insufficiency of Factor VIII is haemophilia A, a sex-linked disease present in males, but female carriers have lowered levels of Factor VIII which may require correction for surgery. Deficiency of Factor IX causes haemophilia B (Christmas disease), seen in males.

Clotting failure may also occur for want of prothrombin, which is formed in the liver, and vitamin K is necessary for its synthesis.

Fibrinolysis

Normal circulating blood contains plasminogen which is the precursor of plasmin, a proteolytic enzyme which breaks down fibrin and fibrinogen and thereby causes the destruction of clots. Though playing a physiological role in the organisation of clots, excessive fibrinolysis can occur in a wide variety of conditions as in sepsis, acute haemorrhage or after major surgery, thus delaying haemostasis.

Table 3.1 Blood clotting process. Note the extrinsic pathway involves few steps and occurs rapidly.

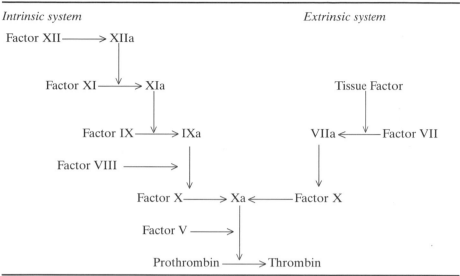

a indicates activated factor.

Von Willebrand's disease

Von Willibrand's factor (VWF) prolongs the life of Factor VIII in the circulation and stabilises platelet plugs. Deficiency affects the level of Factor VIII and platelet function. The disease is seen in males and females.

Anticoagulant therapy

Certain patients will be found who are being treated with anticoagulant drugs following thrombosis or cardiac surgery. Two types of anticoagulant are in use, the rapid and short-acting heparin group which are antithrombins and thereby prevent the conversion of fibrinogen to fibrin, and the longer-acting oral group (such as warfarin), which reduce the amount of circulating prothrombin by preventing its formation in the liver. Patients on anticoagulant therapy should never be taken off these drugs except on a physician's advice. Before surgery is performed the prothrombin time is compared to a control to give the International Normalised Ratio (INR). The therapeutic range is 2.0–4.0. An INR of less than 2.5 is considered safe for most surgery and to achieve this the anticoagulant may have to be stopped for 2 days. The clot may be stabilised with oxidised cellulose (Surgicel).

Liver disease

Many of the factors involved in the clotting cascade are synthesised in the liver and thus any possibility of reduced liver function should be investigated. Cirrhosis of the liver secondary to alcohol abuse may only manifest itself as an

Table 3.2   Relation of factor deficiency and clinical disease.

Factors	Other names	Deficiency disease
Factor I	Fibrinogen	Hypofibrinogenaemia
Factor II	Prothrombin	Hypoprothrombinaemia
Factor III	Thromboplastin	
Factor IV	Calcium ions	
Factor V	Proaccelerin	Factor V deficiency
Factor VI	Does not exist	
Factor VII	Proconvertin	Factor VII deficiency
Factor VIII	Antihaemophilic factor	Haemophilia A
Factor IX	Christmas factor	Haemophilia B
	Plasma thromboplastin component (PTC)	Christmas disease
Factor X	Stuart factor	Stuart factor deficiency
Factor XI	Plasma thromboplastin antecedent (PTA)	PTA deficiency
Factor XII	Hageman factor	Hageman factor deficiency
Factor XIII	Fibrin stabilising factor (FSF)	FSF deficiency

increased tendency to bleed after injury. Careful enquiry should be made as to the patient's alcohol intake. Recent guidelines state that alcohol intake over 28 units per week for a male (21 units per week for a female) is suggestive of alcohol abuse.

Investigation of post-extraction haemorrhage

A history of excessive bleeding is most commonly due to local factors, but particular attention should be paid to those who on several occasions have undergone repeated attempts to arrest post-extraction or other haemorrhage. These need careful investigation to eliminate a possible systemic cause. Petechial haemorrhage (purpura) and bruising are typical of generalised vascular damage and platelet inadequacy, but not of clotting disorders. Recurrent haemarthrosis is suggestive of haemophilia A and B, but not of platelet or vascular disorders. The family history is important as many of the conditions are hereditary.

Wherever the surgeon's suspicions are aroused the patient must be referred to a haematologist for full investigation before operation, as only in the laboratory can the diagnosis be made.

Treatment

Patients with systemic haemorrhagic disease should be admitted to hospital for surgery and treated in conjunction with a haematologist.

In vascular disorders management depends on local measures and arranging for blood to be available for transfusion should *the loss* make this necessary.

In platelet disorders secondary to other diseases the cause must be dealt with first. Patients with idiopathic thrombocytopenia may be given steroid therapy to raise the platelet count or pre-operative platelet infusions.

In clotting disorders the essential treatment is to replace the missing factor. For haemophilia A and Von Willebrand's disease, Factor VIII is available and given by intravenous injection. For patients with mild disease DDAVP (desmopressin) will raise the patient's endogenous Factor VIII. Tranexamic acid is an antifibrinolytic agent used to prevent the destruction of clots and is given for ten days commencing one day pre-operatively.

Choice of anaesthetic

In vascular and platelet disorders either a general or local anaesthetic is satisfactory.

In clotting disorders caution should be used with regard to local anaesthesia, particularly inferior dental and posterior superior dental blocks, owing to the danger of producing a large haematoma which could endanger the airway. Injections down the periodontal membrane may provide adequate anaesthesia for extraction of teeth. General anaesthesia is sometimes indicated and should be administered by an experienced anaesthetist.

Local dental measures

These include oral prophylaxis, improving oral hygiene and *conservation procedures to reduce the number of extractions*. The operation is planned and executed to cause minimal trauma and it is wise to extract teeth from only one quadrant of the mouth at any time. In the local arrest of haemorrhage haemostatic packs such as oxidised cellulose which are bioresorbable may be useful to stabilise the clot.

Respiratory disorders

Bronchitis

This common condition is an acute or chronic inflammation of the mucosa lining the bronchi, which has seasonal exacerbations and is often associated with other conditions, particularly upper respiratory tract infections and bronchiectasis.

All patients suffering from bronchitis and bronchiectasis are best treated under local anaesthesia. Where a general anaesthetic is required they should be assessed by a specialist anaesthetist well beforehand, as many are improved by medical preparation including antibiotics, physiotherapy, and breathing exercises.

Asthma

In asthma there are intermittent attacks of bronchospasm complicated by the secretion of thick mucus and mucosal swelling. It is believed to be an allergic disease, and the use of allergenic substances (e.g. penicillin) is best avoided.

Some patients are under treatment with bronchodilators in the form of an inhaler whilst others may use a corticosteroid aerosol inhaler. General anaesthesia, though not generally contraindicated, should be administered by a specialist anaesthetist.

In acute attacks the airway must be maintained, and in this respect asthmatic patients breathe more easily when upright. To relieve spasm inhalation of the bronchodilator should help, but if this fails, hydrocortisone should be administered intravenously.

Infectious diseases

The dental surgeon and staff are at risk from acquiring infections from patients. These include the common cold, xanthemata, tuberculosis, cytomegalovirus, herpes, hepatitis and human immune deficiency virus (HIV). Precautions must be taken to avoid infection of the surgical team as well as preventing cross-infection between patients.

Viral hepatitis

Several viruses cause hepatitis. Those of importance are virus A, B and C (non-A, non-B). Virus A is transmitted by faecal contamination of food and water and has an incubation period of 30 days. The B virus is transmitted by blood or serum, the incubation period being about 100 days. The virus of hepatitis C has recently been identified and transmission is by blood and serum. Chronic carriers of the hepatitis B – e antigen must be regarded as highly infectious. A very careful operative technique and system for sterilisation of instruments is required to protect surgery staff and other patients. All staff should be advised to be immunised against the hepatitis B virus as unrecognised carriers of the antigen may present for treatment.

Human immune deficiency virus (HIV)

The retrovirus HIV was recognised in 1980 and is transmitted by blood and semen, although it has been isolated from other body fluids. A test for specific antibodies to HIV is available and their presence indicates that the patient can transmit the disease. Whilst some individuals will be aware of their status others may be HIV-positive unknowingly. Since the numbers of affected people is increasing it is wise for precautions to be taken during the treatment of *all* patients, so that there is no risk of infection to the surgical team or other patients. Fortunately the virus is easily inactivated by heat or by the use of hypochlorite.

Those who are HIV-positive are at risk of developing acquired immune deficiency syndrome (AIDS), but the incubation period is unknown. These patients have a compromised cell-mediated immune response and develop opportunistic infections. In the oral cavity candidosis, hairy leukoplakia and Kaposi's sarcoma are manifestations of acquired immune deficiency syndrome. Patients who develop AIDS should be referred to hospital for treatment.

Epilepsy

Epilepsy is a disease of the central nervous system in which there is a paroxysmal electrochemical disturbance. This may result in fits of two types. 'Petit mal' is of a minor character in which, without warning, the patients lose consciousness for a few seconds, but seldom falls or has convulsions. 'Grand mal' is characterised by generalised convulsions and loss of consciousness, and is sometimes heralded by the so-called 'aura', or peculiar sensation, which warns the patient of an impending attack. During the fit the pulse and blood pressure remain normal but muscle contractions may affect respiration causing cyanosis and the tongue may be bitten if not protected.

Prevention is by avoiding excitement and ensuring that patients take their normal dose of anticonvulsant drugs. Where a fit occurs the airway is maintained and the patient turned onto his side and protected from injury. Wooden wedges are inserted between the teeth bilaterally to safeguard the tongue, dentures are removed and the mouth sucked out. Recovery occurs slowly without treatment if the patient is left quietly to regain consciousness. The exception is status epilepticus, where one fit follows another in rapid succession; this may be treated by a slow intravenous injection of diazepam.

Systemic diseases of bone

These conditions affect the dental surgeon in four ways. Difficulties in extraction of teeth may be encountered due to hypercementosis (osteitis deformans – Paget's disease') or sclerosis of bone (osteopetrosis acromegaly). The bone may be fragile, leading to fracture even though minimal force is used during operations (osteogenesis imperfecta). The incidence of post-operative infection is increased (osteitis deformans) and there may be risk of causing an exacerbation of the disease (fibrous dysplasia) or a malignant change in the bone (osteitis deformans).

The successful treatment of these patients lies in a correct diagnosis of the condition followed by careful pre-operative preparation.

Depressive illness

Tricyclic antidepressant drugs which are used in treating depressive illness interact with noradrenaline to cause hypertension but local anaesthetics containing adrenaline appear to be safe. Monoamine oxidase inhibitors are sometimes given for depression. They potentiate the action of many drugs including barbiturates and noradrenaline, the effect lasting for 2 weeks after stopping the drug.

Further reading

Rees, P.J. & Williams, D.G. (1995) *Principles of Clinical Medicine.* Edward Arnold, London.

Spector, T.D. & Axford, J.S. (1999) *An Introduction to General Pathology.* Churchill Livingstone, Edinburgh.

Working Party of the British Society of Antimicrobial Chemotherapy (1997) *Lancet,* 350, 1100.

Chapter 4
Emergencies in Oral Surgery

- Management of collapse
- Fainting
- Anaphylaxis
- Surgical shock
- Acute respiratory obstruction and arrest
- Cardiac arrest
- Cerebral vascular accidents
- Death in the surgery or operating theatre

Any emergency can be terrifying if it occurs without warning and the dental surgeon is unprepared. The element of surprise can be reduced by completing careful histories and investigations to identify the poor-risk patients and enlisting the help of a physician to prepare them for operation. Only by study and experience will the dental surgeon acquire the ability to diagnose and treat quickly those emergencies that may arise. He may be gravely handicapped if the essential drugs and instruments are not readily to hand or if his assistants are untrained.

All essential items for resuscitation should be kept in a special container, the drugs clearly labelled with their name, strength of the solution or tablet, the dose, method of administration and expiry date. Instruments such as hypodermic syringes are stored, ready sterilised, in sealed containers. Oxygen and suction should always be available. Usually two assistants are required, one to help with the patient and one free to fetch and carry. The telephone numbers of the ambulance, fire service, local hospital and the nearest medical practitioners should be readily available.

All these preparations are useless if the team is not regularly rehearsed by mock emergency drills so that each unhesitatingly knows the part he has to play. Emergencies may arise as an acute phase of a known medical condition; this group has been discussed in Chapter 3. Others occur as a result of surgical procedures (Chapter 7) or without previous history, and these are described here.

Management of collapse

- Lay patient flat
- Call for assistance
- Monitor vital signs

- breathing
- pulse
- level of consciousness
- blood pressure
- Initiate treatment as appropriate (CPR etc.)
- If possible ascertain cause of collapse
- Continue monitoring until stable.

Fainting

This is the commonest emergency seen by the dentist as it is often precipitated by the emotional disturbances or pain associated with surgical procedures. In fainting a general peripheral vasodilatation, particularly in the muscles, causes cerebral ischaemia, with loss of consciousness.

Signs and symptoms

These are pallor, nausea, dizziness and a cold sweat, which if ignored are followed by loss of consciousness. The blood pressure falls, the pulse rate remains normal but the volume is weak and thready. The pupils are dilated and rolled up.

Treatment

This consists in promptly lying the patient down in the supine position with the head lower than the heart and the feet well up. The airway is checked, dentures are removed, the jaw is drawn forward and tight clothing is loosened. Verbal communication with the patient is important both as a measure of reassurance and to ascertain their level of consciousness. Starved patients, who are not diabetics, should be given a glucose drink. This treatment is usually successful but should the fall in blood pressure persist oxygen is given and a physician must be consulted.

Anaphylaxis

Anaphylaxis is an acute hypersensitivity reaction to substances to which the patient has been previously sensitised. These may be sera, local anaesthetic solutions, penicillin or other allergenic substances. Prevention is best effected by ensuring that all those with a history of allergy, asthma or hay fever do not receive drugs known to cause such reactions, particularly by injection.

Signs and symptoms

These usually begin within half an hour of introducing the foreign substance. The reaction is characterised by urticaria, particularly at the site of injection, by cyanosis, and dyspnoea due to bronchospasm and oedema, by sweating and a general feeling of faintness. These are accompanied by a raised pulse, a fall in blood pressure and the onset of circulatory collapse and death.

Treatment

This consists in laying the patient down with their feet well up, maintaining the airway and injecting *at once* 0.5–1 ml of adrenaline 1:1,000 solution by intra-muscular injection. This should raise the blood pressure and dilate the bronchi. Where the hypotension persists, a further dose 10 minutes later using a different limb is given. Antihistamine (chlorpheniramine) given by slow intravenous injection may be helpful. The blood pressure is checked repeatedly and if hypotension is persistent an intravenous saline drip may be required.

Hypoglycaemic shock

See Chapter 3.

Acute adrenal insufficiency

See Chapter 3.

Surgical shock

This rarely occurs following oral surgical procedures unless the operation is very prolonged or is accompanied by excessive blood loss. Following severe injury or long continued post-extraction haemorrhage, patients may be seen in a state of shock and require urgent treatment. Surgical shock is a result of fluid loss (either serum from burns or blood from open or closed wounds). In closed wounds blood and plasma may bleed from the vessels into the tissue spaces. It is believed that if the initial loss is over one litre or one quarter of the blood volume of six litres, this is more than can be compensated for by the general vasoconstriction. Where this is not replaced, a vicious circle is set up in which the falling blood pressure and the general vasoconstriction cause oxygen lack in the tissues and an increased permeability of the capillaries with still further loss of fluid into the tissues.

Signs and symptoms

The patient is typically cold, sweating and pale or cyanosed. There is often gasping respiration or air hunger. In the limbs the degree of swelling in closed injuries gives some indication of the fluid loss into the tissues, but this is of little use in facial injuries. The pulse is rapid and the blood pressure low.

Treatment

Prompt and energetic measures in good time are necessary. First, arrest of haemorrhage must be undertaken to prevent further loss, whilst an assistant takes and charts pulse and blood pressure readings at short intervals (15 minutes). In the mildly shocked patient, fluids such as warm, sweet tea may be given by mouth if no operation is envisaged in the next 6 hours, and no abdominal injury is present. A rising pulse rate and a falling blood pressure is an ominous sign. A patient with a pulse rate persistently over 100, and systolic blood pressure of under 100 mm (13.3 KPa), almost certainly requires transfusion and blood should be taken for grouping and cross matching. This should be done early, and whenever there is doubt a slow saline or plasma substitute (e.g. dextran) drip started before the veins collapse.

A choice must be made whether to give saline or plasma to replace fluid, or whole blood which will raise the circulating haemoglobin as well. Unfortunately, haemoglobin estimations are of little use in the acute phase owing to the haemoconcentration which usually occurs. The decision is made from the history or observation of the actual blood loss from open or closed wounds but whichever is given the haemoglobin level must be checked to avoid haemoconcentration or haemodilution.

The circulation to the head is improved by raising the foot of the bed. In cyanosed patients oxygen may be administered. Warmth should be applied with blankets to keep the patient in an environmental temperature of 32°C. No other heating devices, which might cause further peripheral vasodilation, should be used.

Relief of pain may be achieved by temporarily splinting or supporting fractures, by dressing open wounds and by prescribing analgesics.

Acute respiratory obstruction and arrest

This may occur during dental operations under inhalation of general anaesthetic due to the inhalation of vomit or a foreign body if the oro-pharynx is inadequately packed. A second cause is an acute inflammatory swelling of the neck.

Signs and symptoms
The patient stops breathing and though a few jerky respiratory movements are made he is unable to inflate his lungs. The face and neck rapidly become very congested and cyanosed.

Treatment
Immediately the patient becomes anoxic the surgeon should stop the operation, draw the tongue forward, and reduce any pressure from the pack or the chin which might occlude the airway, and suck out any debris in the mouth or oro-pharynx. Meanwhile the anaesthetist searches for any cause of anoxia such as failure of the oxygen supply, obstruction in the tubes of the anaesthetic apparatus, excessive formation of mucus in the respiratory tract, vomiting behind the pack, or swelling of the throat and neck. The dental surgeon should *silently* observe that each has been investigated, but if one is overlooked he should draw attention to it. He should call for the tracheostomy set and can usefully take

the pulse in case cardiac arrest should supervene. The passing of an endotracheal tube will usually restore the airway; however intubation may not be possible, making it necessary to make an opening into the trachea below the obstruction. This may be achieved by cricothyroid puncture or by tracheostomy. These procedures should not be attempted without appropriate training as further damage may occur.

Cricothyroid puncture

A cricothyroid needle, specially designed for the purpose, can be used to pierce the skin and cricothyroid membrane and form a passage for air. However this, though relatively simple to do, can only be considered a temporary expedient.

Emergency tracheostomy

The landmarks for this operation are the cricoid cartilage and the midline of the neck, which may be difficult to identify owing to the gross congestion. The head is held firmly with the neck fully extended over a sandbag so as to bring the trachea as near the surface as possible. The thumb and middle fingers of the left hand palpate and identify the cricoid cartilage which they then grasp throughout the operation (Fig. 4.1).

The incision is made through all the superficial tissues from the thyroid notch to a point one centimetre above the sternal notch. There will be much bleeding

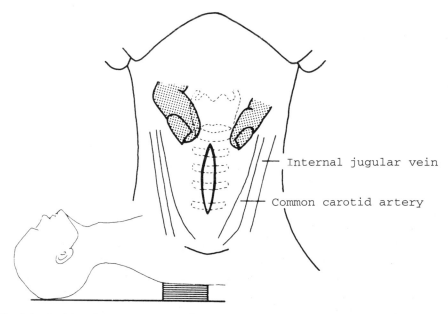

Fig. 4.1 Incision for emergency tracheostomy. Note the position of the thumb, the second finger and major vessels. The first finger has been omitted but enters the wound and palpates the lower border of the cricoid. The inset shows a support under the shoulders to put the neck on full extension.

due to congestion, but if the incision is in the midline, there is no danger. The index finger of the left hand is placed in the wound to identify and protect the cricoid cartilage. The incision is deepened on to the trachea, and the thyroid isthmus is divided if necessary. The second and third tracheal rings are incised. To protect the posterior tracheal wall, all but the last centimetre of the scalpel blade is guarded by gauze or the fingers. The scalpel is withdrawn and the tracheal incision dilated with the handle. Where no introducer or tracheostomy tube is available any rubber tube of about half a centimetre diameter will serve to maintain the airway. Care must be taken that the tube is not accidentally put into the tissues at either side of the trachea. Once the tube is held firmly in place to prevent it displacing into the trachea the emergency is over and respirations should restart and bleeding may be controlled. Once stable the patient should be transferred to an in-patient facility for further management.

Coronary heart disease
See Chapter 3.

Cardiac arrest

Cardiac arrest is of two kinds, cardiac asystole in which the heart is motionless, and ventricular fibrillation in which the action of the heart though present is uncoordinated and ineffective so that circulation is not maintained. The chief predisposing cause is cardiovascular disease and the immediate exciting factors are anoxia, or an overdose of drugs particularly the anaesthetic agent, and vagal stimulation.

Signs and symptoms
The pulse is absent in the carotid and other major arteries, the blood pressure cannot be recorded and bleeding stops from the operation wound. The respirations cease and the pupils are widely dilated and fixed. It must be remembered that the patient's best chance of survival rests in rapid transfer to a centre where specialist resuscitation facilities are available and there should be no delay in calling for help in this situation.

Treatment
Cardiac massage is the only accepted remedy and every dental surgeon must be prepared to attempt it *without delay*; three minutes is the limit of anoxia that the brain will tolerate before irreversible changes take place. The anaesthetist (or the surgeon's assistant if the arrest occurs under local anaesthetic) lays the patient flat and maintains a clear airway by removing all obstructions, drawing the tongue forward and pushing the jaw forward by pressing at the angles. He insufflates the lungs, preferably using oxygen through an endotracheal tube or a face mask and ventilating bag. Where these are not available mouth-to-mouth breathing may be used.

Mouth to mouth respiration

After clearing the mouth and pharynx of debris and fluids, the neck is extended by flexing the head dorsally. The chin is drawn forward by grasping the lower jaw with one hand, whilst the other pinches the nostrils to seal them. The operator's wide open mouth is applied to the patient's (or an airway) to form an airtight seal. Air is then exhaled into the patient's mouth with sufficient force and volume to expand his lungs. The chest should be seen to rise and fall between each breath. This is repeated 12 to 18 times a minute. Where available a Brook airway or Laerdal pocket mask will facilitate artificial respiration.

Cardiac massage

The surgeon strips the patient's chest of all clothing preparatory to giving cardiac massage. External cardiac massage is given by lying the patient flat on a firm surface. The operator kneels beside him and places the palm of one hand on the sternum just above the xiphisternum. The other hand is laid over the first. The arms are kept straight and with the whole weight of the body the sternum is depressed about 5 cm downwards (Fig. 4.2). In this way the heart is compressed between the sternum and the vertebral column and the ventricles

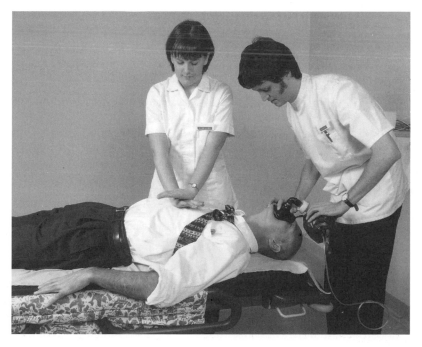

Fig. 4.2 Cardio pulmonary resuscitation (CPR). Note use of mask and bag connected to oxygen.

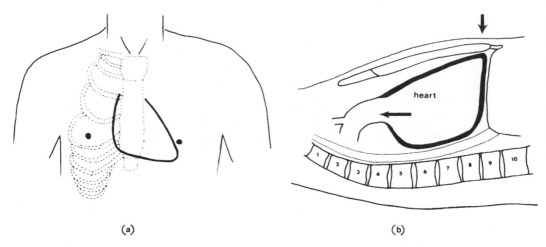

(a)   (b)

Fig. 4.3   (a) Shows the relationship of the heart to the sternum and ribs. (b) Shows how pressure on the xiphisternum compresses the heart between the sternum and the vertebral column.

empty (Fig. 4.3). Pressure is reapplied in this way 60 to 80 times a minute and if done satisfactorily a circulation can be maintained with a recordable blood pressure. In children the pressure should be less and applied to the middle of the sternum at a rate of 100 times a minute.

To allow effective ventilation, insufflation is performed at every fifth *upstroke* of cardiac massage. Where one individual is faced with both tasks he will similarly insufflate the lungs twice between each fifteen strokes of cardiac massage. About ten minutes of this exercise is as much as one person can manage but massage should normally be continued till the heart starts beating normally or expert help, with a defibrillator, is available.

If vital signs are restored, the patient should be turned into the recovery position (Fig. 4.4) while monitoring continues.

Cerebral vascular accidents

An acute cerebral vascular accident may occur as a result of rupture, thrombosis or embolism in a cerebral vessel.

Signs and symptoms

These will obviously vary widely according to the size and the site of the vessels involved. The following are typical of most such catastrophes. The onset is sudden but not all patients go into coma. The face is flushed or cyanosed, breathing slow and stertorous and the pulse is slow and bounding. Hemiplegia and changes in reactions of the pupils are frequently present. In conscious patients the speech is often affected.

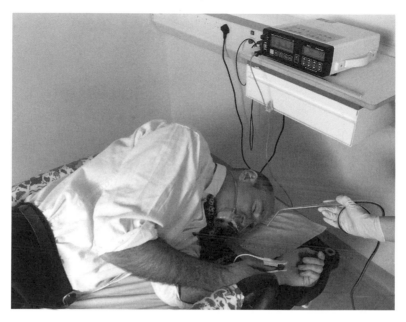

Fig. 4.4 Recovery position. Suction, oxygen and monitoring equipment should be readily available.

Treatment

This consists of maintaining the airway and giving oxygen. The patient should be kept quiet and not moved till seen by a physician.

Death in the surgery or operating theatre

When death occurs the dental surgeon should tell the patient's relatives and general medical practitioner, speaking to the relatives personally. The coroner must be notified as soon as possible of the name and address of the deceased and the time and circumstances of the death. A written report must be submitted to the coroner's clerk within 24 hours. The dental surgeon may attend the post-mortem if it is ordered and it is advisable to do so. He may be directed, by the coroner, to attend the inquest and give evidence. It is wise in the case of such a calamity to seek the advice of a medical protection society before writing the report or attending the post-mortem or inquest.

Further reading

Colquhoun, M., Handley, A.J., Evans, T.R. & Resus Council (UK) (1999) *ABC of Resuscitation*, 4th edn. BMJ Publishing Group, London.

Jones, R.D.M. & Holland, R.B. (1997) *Anaesthesia and Resuscitation: a houseman's guide*. Butterworth Heinemann, Oxford.

Chapter 5
Pharmacology and Oral Surgery

- Pre-operative medication
- Peri-operative medication
- Post-operative medication
- Traumatic injuries
- Infections
- Medication of packs for sockets

The successful practice of oral surgery depends on the use of certain drugs. Principally these are medications involved in the management of pain and anxiety and in control of infection. These drugs may be:

- Administered by the dentist or oral surgeon
- Recommended for purchase over the counter by the dentist
- Prescribed by the dentist

Many drugs which the dentist can prescribe (such as aspirin and paracetamol) are cheaper when bought over the counter. When prescribing a drug it is important to consider the following points.

The pharmacological action of the drug

At no time should any drug be prescribed if its action is not clearly understood. In this respect side-effects should be carefully considered. The British National Formulary, published twice-yearly, gives a good outline of action and side effects and should be consulted if there is any doubt about the suitability of a particular drug. It is a good principle to have a repertoire of a few well-tried drugs which meet the needs of day-to-day practice, and to understand them well, rather than to experiment with a wide range.

Contraindications and incompatibility of drugs

In certain medical conditions some drugs are contraindicated, for example aspirin in severe renal disease. Incompatibility of drugs only arises occasionally, though it should be borne in mind, but a more common and dangerous complication is an anaphylactic reaction in those patients sensitive to a drug (e.g. penicillin). It is therefore important to question the patient carefully about previous treatment and reaction and any history of urticaria or asthma, as sufferers from these conditions seem more likely to be sensitive. Wherever there is doubt about the proposed drug an alternative should be used.

Dosage

Today the formularies make it unnecessary to give details of the constituent parts of medicines, but the correct title and strength of the drug, together with the four 'Hows' must be clearly stated:

- *How much* of the drug is to be taken in each individual dose
- *How often* it is to be taken, expressed as the number of doses in each 24 hours and the interval between each
- *How long* the course is to run, expressed in days, so that it is not continued overlong or stopped before the clinician thinks fit
- *How* it is to be administered, by mouth, intramuscularly, etc.

The British National Formularies give suggested doses of accepted remedies for adults and children, to which reference should be made before prescribing. Excretion of drugs in the elderly may be slow and particular care is needed when prescribing drugs for them.

The importance of giving adequate doses for a specific purpose cannot be overstressed. Low doses must be avoided if drug therapy is to be effective.

An example of wording on a prescription is shown here:

Date

Rx   250 mg phenoxymethyl penicillin tablets
Send 20 (twenty)
Label 1 tablet orally 4 times daily for 5 days.

Signature

Methods of administration

The routes of administration of a drug are divided into enteral and parenteral. Enteral routes are gastro-intestinal and include:

- Oral
- Sublingual
- Rectal

Parenteral modes of administration are:

- Topical
- Inhalational

- By injection
- By intravenous infusion

Dentists may use some of these routes to administer drugs. The timing of the administration of drugs can be divided into:

- Pre-operative
- Peri-operative
- Post-operative

Pre-operative medication

Pre-operative drugs may be used for the following reasons:

- Anxiolysis
- Pre-emptive analgesia
- Prophylaxis to prevent infection

Anxiolysis

The most commonly used drugs at present for reduction of anxiety prior to surgical treatments are the benzodiazepines. When used in this regard these drugs are taken orally. In addition to producing anxiolysis these agents are also hypnotics and thus can ensure a good night's sleep prior to surgery. Commonly used preparations for anxiolysis are diazepam and temazepam. Nitrazepam is a good hypnotic. In children chloral hydrate may be useful.

Pre-emptive analgesia

Post-operative pain is a consequence of many surgical procedures and operations performed in the mouth and jaws are no exception. The initiators of the pain process are produced by tissue damage. Therefore it is sensible to obtain adequate plasma levels of analgesic drugs at the time of tissue damage. Thus analgesics should begin prior to surgery. Non-steroidals such as ibuprofen taken 40 minutes orally before surgery or diclofenac administered per rectum in those having general anaesthesia should be considered.

Some operators prescribe corticosteroids pre-operatively in an attempt to reduce post-operative swelling. In some instances this is legitimate; however, for routine surgical procedures such as the removal of impacted third molar teeth it is probably unwarranted.

Infection prophylaxis

The use of antibiotics prior to oral surgical procedures may be used to prevent infection of the surgical wound or of a distant site (such as damaged heart valves). Wound infection is not common after oral surgical procedures and thus antibiotics are not routinely prescribed. The indications for the use of prophylactic antibiotics to prevent wound infection are:

- In a patient with reduced host resistance
- When inserting foreign material (implants)
- Transplantation of teeth
- For procedures lasting longer than 2 hours

When prescribing antibiotics for the prevention of wound infection it is important to administer a bactericidal antibiotic at the correct dose at the correct time. Maximal plasma levels of the drug should be present at the time the blood clot is forming. This is achieved by administering at least twice the normal therapeutic dose orally 1 hour before clot formation is anticipated, or IV at the end of the procedure. A single dose is sufficient. The use of antibiotics to *prevent* wound infection after clot formation has occurred does not make sense. A suitable drug for use in wound prophylaxis is amoxycillin; in those allergic to penicillin a single dose of clindamycin is an alternative.

When administering antibiotics to prevent distant infection such as infective endocarditis the timing is different to that discussed above. In this case the aim is to achieve sufficient drug concentration at the *start* of the procedure. Thus when administering drugs orally they would be given one hour before the operation commences. Table 5.1 gives the recommended prophylactic regimens at the time of writing for the prevention of infective endocarditis.

Peri-operative medication

Sedative and anaesthetic drugs are used to allow the successful practice of oral surgery. The use of general anaesthesia for minor oral surgical procedures in adults should be discouraged. Nevertheless this form of anaesthesia is still required for major procedures and for some minor operations in young children. Indeed, even in children the use of sedation permits the carrying out of operations which previously were performed under general anaesthesia.

Intravenous sedation

The drug of choice in adults at present is the benzodiazepine midazolam, although other drugs such as propofol are used in some centres.

Midazolam is administered intravenously in 1.0 mg increments every minute until a state of sedation is reached. The average dose for sedation is in the range 0.07–0.1 mg/kg. Local anaesthetic may then be administered. When performing intravenous sedation a second appropriately trained person must be present throughout the procedure, and adequate chaperoning of the patient must be

Table 5.1   Prevention of endocarditis (adult doses*).

Drug Regimens		Dose	Route	Time (hours)
Under local anaesthesia				
Either	Amoxycillin	3 g	oral	−1
or	Clindamycin	600 mg	oral	−1
Under general anaesthesia				
Either	Amoxycillin	1 g	IV	at induction
		500 mg	oral	+6
or	Amoxycillin	3 g	oral	−4
		3 g	oral	post-op
*Special risk**				
Either	Amoxycillin	1 g	IV	at induction
	Gentamicin	120 mg	IV	at induction
	Amoxycillin	500 mg	oral	+6
or	Vancomycin	1 g	IV infusion	−1.5
	Gentamicin	120 mg	IV	at induction
or	Teicoplanin	400 mg	IV	at induction
	Gentamicin	120 mg	IV	at induction
or	Clindamycin	300 mg	IV infusion	at induction
	Clindamycin	150 mg	IV/oral	+6

* Children under 10 receive 50% of the adult dose; those under 5 receive 25% of the adult dose (except for vancomycin where children receive 20 mg/kg, teicoplanin where the dose is 6 mg/kg and gentamicin where the dose is 2 mg/kg).
** Patients with a history of infective endocarditis; patients with prosthetic heart valves requiring general anaesthesia; patients allergic to or having received penicillin in the previous month and requiring general anaesthesia.

arranged. Monitoring the patient's responses both visually and mechanically is essential when performing intravenous sedation; the use of a pulse oximeter is considered essential. Oxygen, adequate suction equipment and the benzodiazepine reversal agent flumazenil must be at hand. Intravenous sedation with midazolam provides between 30 minutes and 1 hour of sedation and this is ideal for many oral surgery procedures. In addition to the sedative properties of midazolam it is an excellent amnesic drug. Patients must be advised prior to the sedation appointment that on the day of surgery they should not drive, operate machinery or sign important legal documents. In addition an appropriate adult must accompany them home after they are sedated.

Inhalation sedation (relative analgesia)

Although inhalation sedation is used in adults for oral surgery it is more commonly employed in children. In addition to producing sedation the mixture of nitrous oxide and oxygen produces a degree of pain control in its own right (hence the name relative analgesia). In this technique the gaseous mixture is inhaled via a nasal mask and the concentration of nitrous oxide in the mixture slowly increased until an appropriate level of sedation is achieved. Usually the concentration of nitrous oxide in the inhaled gas is in the range 30–50%. The use of inhalation sedation in combination with local anaesthesia allows the performance of procedures in children which previously were carried out under general anaesthesia.

Local anaesthesia

Local anaesthetic drugs may be used to reduce operative pain either alone or in combination with sedation or general anaesthesia. The use of local anaesthesia during general anaesthesia offers a number of advantages. These include:

- Reduced dose of general anaesthetic
- Operative haemostasis
- Reduced post-operative pain
- Reduced post-operative analgesic intake

When used alone for operative procedures local anaesthetics can be used:

- Topically
- As infiltration anaesthesia
- As regional block anaesthesia
- As intra-osseous (including intraligamentary) anaesthesia

The gold standard local anaesthetic is 2% lidocaine with epinephrine. This provides reliable anaesthesia following injection and provides good haemostasis. The concentration of epinephrine varies in different parts of the world (in the UK 1:80000 is the standard; in other countries 1:200000 is used). The maximum dose of lidocaine is 4.4 mg/kg. When epinephrine has to be avoided the alternative vasoconstrictor is felypressin which is supplied in combination with the local anaesthetic agent prilocaine (3% prilocaine with 0.03 IU/ml felypressin). The maximum dose of prilocaine is 6.0 mg/kg. If a vasoconstrictor-free solution must be used (for example if local vascularity is severely compromised after therapeutic irradiation) then 4% prilocaine plain or 3% mepivacaine are the solutions of choice. The maximum dose of mepivacaine is 4.4 mg/kg.

When performing surgical procedures which produce significant post-operative pain the use of a long-acting local anaesthetic should be considered. Drugs such as bupivacaine can produce long-lasting anaesthesia (6–8 hours) when administered as a regional block. Bupivacaine is available as 0.25% and 0.5% solutions plain and with epinephrine at a dose of 1:200000. The maximum dose of bupivacaine is 1.3 mg/kg.

Post-operative medication

Post-operative problems following oral surgery include pain, swelling, trismus and (if a general anaesthetic has been used) nausea. Some of these problems can be prevented by pre-emptive medication and a careful surgical technique. However post-operative analgesic medication is usual after some procedures.

Post-operative analgesia

Most of the pain caused by oral surgery is inflammatory in nature. Therefore analgesic drugs with an anti-inflammatory action are recommended. The mainstays of post-operative analgesia therapy are non-steroidal anti-inflammatory drugs such as aspirin, ibuprofen and diclofenac. In patients who cannot take this type of medication paracetamol is the second choice. Patients should be advised to take analgesics following surgery as a routine if that particular procedure is known to produce pain. Third molar surgery for example can produce significant pain for three days after surgery, therefore patients having this procedure should be prepared to take analgesics for this time and not wait for the discomfort to occur.

Post-operative vomiting

Nausea may occur after a general anaesthetic and this can be controlled by the use of an intravenous anti-emetic medication such as ondansetron or the intramuscular agent prochlorperazine. Although oral anti-emetic preparations are available their use in the control of post-operative vomiting is unlikcly to be successful.

Traumatic injuries

Analgesics and hypnotics

In traumatic injuries these may be prescribed as necessary provided the patient's reflexes are not so depressed that the airway may obstruct from bleeding or other causes. Similarly in a suspected head injury opiate analgesics or sedative drugs which could mask the signs of progressive intracranial pressure are to be avoided. All drugs given to patients must be carefully recorded and if the patient is transferred elsewhere the record must be sent with them.

Anti-infectives

Antibacterial substances are used prophylactically for a few days where there is a large haematoma which may become infected, and for a longer period where the deeper tissues, and particularly bone, have been contaminated.

In maxillary fractures which involve the cranial fossae with loss of cerebro-spinal fluid through the nose, ears or pharynx, it is important to prevent intracranial infection by the use of an antibacterial which will cross the thecal barrier.

In all penetrating wounds contaminated with road dirt or soil the need for tetanus prophylaxis must be considered. In patients who have not been immunised or where 10 years have elapsed since the last reinforcing dose, 0.5 ml of absorbed tetanus vaccine should be given by intramuscular injection.

Infections

Today antibacterial drugs play an important part in the treatment of acute infections but they should not be considered a substitute for necessary surgery, though they are useful as a preparation or adjunct to such treatment. The object is to select for use the agent which gives the best therapeutic result with the minimal side effects. To do this the condition must be diagnosed, the causal organism isolated and its susceptibility to antibacterials tested *in vitro* (see Chapter 12). A course is then planned of sufficient concentration and duration that the formation of resistant strains is prevented. A satisfactory concentration in the blood is obtained by administering the drug parenterally wherever possible, and a high initial 'loading' dose is to be recommended. The drug should be changed if there is no response after 48 hours. Generally the agents of choice are penicillin, amoxycillin, flucloxacillin and metronidazole. Where necessary, erythromycin and clindamycin are used. Combinations of antibacterial drugs must be used with caution. Some combinations are effective, for example penicillin and metronidazole.

On many occasions, where it is not possible to ascertain the sensitivity of the organism, it may be essential to prescribe blind, but it should never be regarded as the method of choice. An antibiotic known to be effective in the type of infection under consideration should be used. In oral surgery this is commonly a penicillin, but if there is no response after 48 hours another antibacterial should be selected.

Medication of packs for sockets

It is often necessary to dress bone cavities after oral surgery. The two medicaments most frequently used on ribbon gauze are bismuth, iodoform and paraffin paste (BIPP) or Whitehead's varnish (iodoform 200 g, benzoin 200 g, storax 150 g, balsam of tolu 100 g in ether to 2l). BIPP may give rise to toxic symptoms from absorption of the bismuth but this is most unusual on small packs in sockets though it may occur if used on large packs in big cavities. Whitehead's varnish contains iodoform and patients may be sensitive to this, but it is otherwise safe and widely used. Custom-designed medications such as Alvogyl, which contains a topical anaesthetic, and iodoform and eugenol may also be used to treat 'dry socket'.

In addition to local treatments the use of non-steroidal anti-inflammatory drugs should be recommended to alleviate the discomfort of this painful condition.

Adverse drug reactions

Occasionally a patient will report an unexpected adverse reaction to a drug or medicament. In an attempt to identify such problems at an early stage, a system of individual reporting of occurrences has been developed. The Committee on Safety of Medicines (CSM) collates the information and suitable forms for reporting will be found in the British National Formulary.

Further reading

British National Formulary, current edition (produced biannually). Pharmaceutical Press, London.

Seymour, R.A., Meechan, J.G. & Yates, M.S. (1999) *Pharmacology and Dental Therapeutics*, 3rd edn. Oxford University Press, Oxford.

Chapter 6
The Operating Room, Instruments and the Surgical Team

- The operating room
- Equipment
- Instruments
- Sterilisation
- The surgical team
- Sterile technique
- The operation
- The close of the operation

This chapter discusses the dental surgery or theatre, the instruments for oral surgical operations and the preparation of the surgical team.

The operating room

The operating room both in hospital and general dental practice should be of simple design, the walls and furniture of materials easy to clean and the equipment normally required accommodated without overcrowding.

It should be well ventilated and kept at an even temperature of 18–21°C, without undue humidity. In hospital theatres this is best done by positive pressure air-conditioning which also prevents contamination from the outside atmosphere. Next door to the operating room there should be a central recovery room with experienced nursing staff where the patient may recover on a couch or trolley within easy reach of surgeon and anaesthetist until both are satisfied that he is fit to return to the ward or to go home.

Equipment

Light

The light source should provide adequate illumination without production of heat, and be easily adjusted to shine into the mouth. A headlamp or fibre light attached to a handpiece are recommended for operations involving the palate or deep cavities such as cysts or the antrum.

Suction apparatus

No procedure however minor, particularly under general anaesthesia, should be attempted without suction apparatus. This must be tested before the operation starts and whenever possible an alternative form of suction should be available in case of breakdown. Electrical apparatus is very powerful but does occasionally fail. Suction from the water supply is very effective, simple, trouble-free and economical, and is ideally suited to the dental surgery. Compressed air can also provide powerful suction in a similar way. Whichever method is used a catchment bottle must be included in the circuit so that if roots are lost the bottle may be searched.

Radiographic viewing box

This should be so placed that the dental surgeon can see it without moving from the dental chair or operating table. It should incorporate a spotlight.

The dental engine

Though the conventional dental handpiece can be sterilised, its attachment to the dental electric engine or air motor presents a problem. The surgeon may be contaminated from the cable drive unless this is covered with a sterile sleeve. Alternatively, sterilisable surgical motors and handpieces are available, but due to their high cost these are usually only found in hospital practice. For the clean and rapid cutting of the bone without overheating it is necessary that the bur be washed by a continuous stream of sterile water. Handpieces with an integral irrigation system are available and provide automatic irrigation of the bur. The air-rota is not advocated for oral surgery due to the risk of contamination of the wound with oil and the introduction of air into the tissues to cause surgical emphysema. The modern electrical motor gives very adequate speed and torque.

The dental chair

This should be of a design in which the patient can lie flat and the operator may work seated as this is the position of choice. The light, dental engine and suction should be sufficiently adjustable that they can be used with a supine patient from either right or left side.

Electrical equipment

Where this is to be used in the presence of anaesthetic vapours which may form explosive mixtures of gases, the equipment, particularly the dental engine, must be adequately sealed and earthed by a competent electrician to prevent sparking or a build-up of static electricity which might cause an explosion.

Lasers

Modern lasers give excellent control for dissection of soft tissues. Cells in the path of the cut are vapourised with little damage on either side. Their principle advantage in excisions in the mouth is the relatively small amount of post-operative pain, and a reduction in tissue swelling. Stringent safety measures must be taken during the use of the equipment to avoid damage to the patient and the operators. Laserproof glasses should be worn by all personnel in theatre at all times when the laser is in use to protect the eyes. The endo-tracheal tube should also be protected to avoid inadvertent puncture and metal instruments should be avoided to decrease possible reflection of the beam.

Cryotherapy

Cryosurgery using liquid nitrous oxide, carbon dioxide, or nitrogen destroys cells by intracellular ice crystal formation which ruptures the cell membrane. Healing of the tissue damage is by regeneration of normal tissue. It is of particular benefit in the treatment of benign soft tissue lesions and fluid filled lesions such as haemangiomas.

Operating microscope

This is essential equipment for micro-vascular surgery and nerve repair. Up to 40× magnification is possible.

Instruments

The selection of hand instruments depends on the surgeon's preference. In the succeeding chapters instruments suitable for the various procedures are suggested. It is the surgeon's responsibility to check that all those he needs are readily available. They should be laid up on sterile towels on a trolley.

Care and maintenance of surgical instruments

The principles of care and maintenance are four: to clean the instruments thoroughly, to examine them for defects, to repair or discard those that are defective, and to sharpen all cutting edges.

Mechanical cleaning

Mucus and clotted blood may harbour and protect bacteria and make it impossible for steam to reach them. The first step in the process of sterilisation is to scrub all instruments until clean with a brush under a running cold water tap. A bath agitated by ultrasonic vibrations produces a very high standard of cleanliness especially for hinged instruments and for suction tubes and heads. The latter should have cold water sucked through them immediately the operation is finished.

Cleaning also includes stripping down, cleaning and oiling all working machinery such as handpieces.

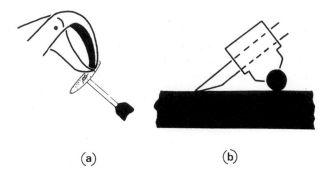

(a) (b)

Fig. 6.1 Sharpening of instruments: (a) sandpaper disc for sharpening *outside* of forceps blade; (b) chisel held at the correct angle on the stone by a hone guide.

Examination for defects

Broken or bent instruments are put aside for repair or discarded. Hinges are tightened if necessary. Disposable items, burs, injection needles and scalpel blades are thrown away.

Sharpening

Stainless steel forceps and elevators are sharpened with a sandpaper disc in the dental handpiece (Fig. 6.1). It is only used on the outside of the blades, care being taken to maintain the angle of manufacture. There is a limit to how often these instruments can be sharpened before the working ends become too short.

Chisels have two bevels, one for grinding and one for sharpening. The angle for grinding is 20–25° and for sharpening 35°. Grinding is best left to an instrument technician and is done infrequently. Sharpening must be done each time the chisel is used. A hone guide will hold the bevelled side at the correct angle to the oil-stone when rubbing it up. Finally the flat side of the chisel is laid on the stone and rubbed two or three times to smooth the edge.

Sterilisation

- Kills all microorganisms
- Chemical or physical methods are used
- Steam at high pressure (autoclave)
- Boiling water only disinfects

Physical and chemical methods are both in use today. Physical methods include wet and dry heat, and gamma radiation (used commercially for sterilising packed instruments such as scalpel blades). Boiling water is no longer regarded as a safe method of sterilisation as it only disinfects and does not kill sporing organisms.

Autoclaves use steam under pressure. Some are high vacuum but all depend on downward displacement of air by steam. Steam at $2\,kg/cm^2$ pressure gives a temperature of 134°C which in 3 minutes will destroy all organisms and spores. It is the method of choice for dressing and towels, but they must be packed loosely to allow the steam to circulate. Blunting of instruments is due to oxidation which should not occur in a properly functioning autoclave, so it can be safely used for sharp instruments. Vapour phase inhibitor (VPI) paper can be used to wrap instruments such as burs which tend to rust if autoclaved. Handpieces must be cleaned and oiled before being placed in the autoclave. The oil must not become oxidised or lose its oily properties at high temperatures.

Dry heat is effective in ovens which have fans to ensure even heat distribution and a door-lock which prevents opening during the sterilising period. The cycle is much slower as it takes half an hour at 160°C to destroy organisms and spores. It may be used for sharp instruments and handpieces. Both autoclaves and hot-air sterilisers are made with controlled cycles which cannot be interrupted once started so that sterility of the instruments is ensured. The efficiency of the cycle must be checked periodically by the use of Brownes' tubes.

Chemical sterilising is not regarded favourably by bacteriologists as most of the solutions available are not considered reliable. Glutaraldehyde is effective against vegetative organisms and spores if the instruments are immersed in it for ten hours, after which it must be washed off with sterile water, as it is irritant to tissues. Because of the length of the sterilising time and the irritant properties the use of glutaraldehyde is confined to those instruments which cannot be heat sterilised. Glutaraldehyde or hypochlorite solutions may be used to disinfect instruments potentially heavily contaminated with viruses (such as hepatitis) before these are cleaned and sterilised.

Both gamma radiation and ethylene oxide are used commercially for the sterilisation of disposables such as scalpel blades and sutures but their toxicity precludes their use in the surgery.

To sterilise with certainty autoclaving is the method of choice. Dry heat sterilising is the next best and only where both of these are impossible should chemical sterilising be considered.

Instruments packs

In hospital practice instruments are sterilised wrapped in paper containers. These are permeable to the steam in the autoclave and, providing the latter is of an evacuating type, are dry at the end of the cycle. Packs may be made up of one instrument or a complete layout for an operation including towels. They can be stored for up to six months ready for immediate use. The packs are duplicated according to the frequency with which they are used and may be prepared for local anaesthetic injections, flap preparation, suturing and so forth. This system is seldom available in general dental practice, making it necessary to sterilise and lay up instruments for each operation separately, though the hot air oven does make it possible to put groups of instruments in metal boxes which can then be stored sterile.

The surgical team

- Surgeon
- Anaesthetist
- Assistant
- Nursing staff

The surgeon

The surgeon is responsible for checking the identity of the patient and the nature of the operation to be performed, for the operation and for the surgical safety of the patient. His whole attention and effort must be devoted to this task and every assistance given him, that it may be completed safely and well. He is answerable for any procedure, planned or accidental, inflicted on the patient including those carried out by his assistants. He must be satisfied that all instruments swabs and packs are accounted for at the end of the operation.

All experienced staff realise the responsibility that rests on the surgeon and will overlook minor breaches of self-control that may occur. However, in an emergency, where speed and efficiency are wanted, an equable temperament and a firm determined manner will be more effective than any amount of histrionics.

The anaesthetist

The anaesthetist assesses the patient's fitness for general anaesthesia, chooses the anaesthetic agent, prescribes suitable premedication and administers the general anaesthetic. He will supervise the moving of the patient to and from the ward, and on and off the operating table, as well as his recovery from the anaesthetic and such post-anaesthetic complications as may arise.

During the operation he is responsible for the patient's airway, which should include packing of the throat and the removal of the pack after operation. He should continually assess the patient's general condition and report any deterioration to the surgeon, so that a mutual assessment of the situation can be made. The anaesthetist's opinion about the safety of the patient is accepted and surgical procedures planned or modified accordingly.

The surgeon's assistant

The oral surgeon's assistant in the hospital theatre is either a qualified colleague (house-surgeon or registrar) or a member of the nursing staff. In the dental surgery it will usually be a dental nurse who, when trained by the dental surgeon, can be most efficient. The assistant will produce the patient's notes and radiographs and mount the latter correctly on the viewing box. He will then help with the preparation of the patient, by cleaning and towelling up the operation area and assembling the suction and other dental apparatus.

He will retract the tissues to give the surgeon the best possible access, clear fluid from the field of the operation with suction or swabs and remove solid debris with forceps. He assists with haemostasis by applying pressure or artery forceps, and with suturing by cutting the ends of the sutures.

The longer two people work together the greater will be the degree of teamwork possible, with mutual benefit to all concerned. The surgeon will ask for further help in various special ways and, from qualified staff, advice based on previous experience, thereby extending their field of interest and responsibility.

The nursing staff

Before the operation begins the nursing staff will select and lay up those instruments, drugs and dressings they know to be necessary. They check the working of the dental engine and suction apparatus, and of all electrical appliances.

They follow the progress of the operation closely in order to anticipate the surgeon's needs and inspect and clean instruments, drawing attention to any that become broken or damaged. At the beginning and at the end of the operation they count all swabs, packs, dressings, instruments and needles, and tell the surgeon if any are missing before the patient leaves the theatre or the outpatient surgery.

Preparation of the surgical team

Those taking part in a surgical operation must be free from infection, especially of the respiratory tract or skin, which could be transmitted to the wound. All are responsible for their own safety and must develop a sensible routine which avoids skin or conjunctiva from being contaminated by blood or saliva from patients.

Sterile technique

- Minimising contamination of the wound
- Wearing 'scrubs' and clogs
- Scrubbing up
- Sterile gowns and gloves
- Sterile instruments
- Preparing operation site with antiseptic solution
- Avoiding contamination during surgery

Dress

All those entering a hospital operating theatre must change from their normal clothes into freshly laundered drill trousers and shirt, or dresses. This not only reduces the risk of contamination but is cooler and more comfortable, The hair is covered with a paper cap and a mask is worn over the mouth and nose. Safety glasses should be worn to avoid splashing of blood or irrigation fluid into the eyes. Shoes are changed for antistatic pumps, rubber boots or clogs used only in the theatre.

In the dental surgery a freshly laundered gown worn over everyday clothes is put on for each patient. A mask and protective glasses should be worn. The use of a cap is optional.

Scrubbing up

Those who have to handle sterile instruments or dressings must undertake the ritual of 'scrubbing up'. The arms are bared to the elbow and all rings and watches removed. The hands and forearms are washed under a running tap, using an antiseptic detergent solution. They are well soaped and washed from the tips of the fingers up towards the elbow. The fingernails must be kept trimmed short for satisfactory cleansing which is done with a sterile scrubbing brush or nail scraper. At intervals, but not too frequently, the suds are rinsed away under the tap, being made to flow off at the elbow, not at the hands. This is continued for 4 minutes by the clock. The hands are then dried on a sterile towel by wiping from the hands up to the elbows. For minor procedures carried out in the dental surgery sterile gloves are put on and the operation commenced. For more extensive operations or where there is a risk of infection of staff and in theatre to conform with normal practice, a sterile gown and gloves are worn.

Gowning up

The sterile gown is lifted from its container folded in such a way that if held correctly with both hands at its neck, it will unroll and fall with the sleeves hanging away from the operator. The arms are then placed in the sleeves and a second person standing behind draws the gown over the shoulders and fastens the tapes and belt at the back. The belt avoids billowing and rubbing of the gown and is an antistatic precaution.

Surgical gloves are then put on. There is now a large selection on the market to cater for all aspects of surgery. Powder free gloves are now the norm and alternatives for those who are latex sensitve are becoming available. The gloves are taken from their envelope by the cuffs, which are folded down over the palms. The cuff of the right glove is held in the left hand and the right hand thrust in. The right hand then lifts the left glove by placing the fingers *under* the rolled cuff and the left hand is thrust in. The cuffs are turned back over the wrist to cover the sleeve. In this way at no time will the hands have been in contact with outside of either gown or gloves. From this moment if any unsterilised object is touched the operator must gown up again.

An alternative method had been introduced to reduce the risk of contamination of the outside of the gown or gloves. After gowning, both hands remain

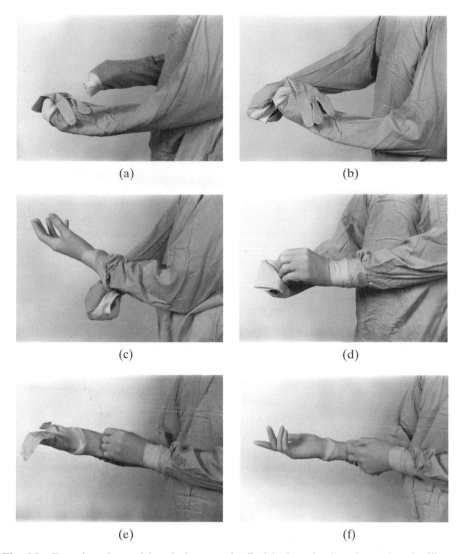

Fig. 6.2 Donning gloves (closed glove method): (a) glove is placed over hand still within gown, fingers pointing up arm; (b) cuff of glove is grasped through gown by left and right hand, glove is pulled over left hand; (c) left hand is then thrust into glove; (d) left hand then positions glove on right hand; (e) and pulls glove over hand while; (f) hand emerges from gown into glove.

covered by the sleeves. The left glove, with its fingers directed towards the elbow, is placed with the palm surface against the left sleeve. The cuff of the glove is grasped through the material by the thumb and fingers of the left hand. The right hand (through the gown material) grasps the outer part of the glove cuff and turns it over the sleeve of the gown. The glove is drawn onto the left hand by pulling glove and sleeve up the forearm (Fig. 6.2).

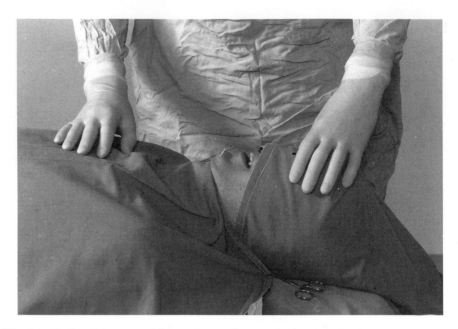

Fig. 6.3   Patient is protected by sterile towels to reduce contamination.

Preparation of the patient

In hospitals a label carrying the patient's name, address and hospital number is attached to the wrist. The details should be checked against the patient's notes. A valid consent form must be available before the general anaesthetic is started. When local anaesthetic is being used mistaken idenity may be avoided by direct questioning of the patient.

In theatre with the patient lying on the operating table, intubated and with the throat packed off, the surgeon checks his position on the table and has it adjusted if unsatisfactory. The operator then cleanses the site of operation, usually the mouth and surrounding skin, with a swab held in forceps and dipped in a detergent (chlorhexidine), care being taken to protect the eyes. The patient's body and head are then covered with sterile towels in such a way as to leave only the operation site exposed (Fig. 6.3). For extraoral procedures the mouth is also covered.

In the out-patient surgery the patient should be asked to wash the mouth thoroughly with a mouth wash and in the case of female patients all cosmetics should be removed. A sterile towel may then be pinned round the patient's neck and a sterile cap placed over the hair, to prevent contamination of the instruments or of the operator's hands. The patient's eyes are protected from the light and instruments by dark glasses.

The operation

All members of the team must work in a comfortable position to avoid fatigue. Modern equipment makes it possible for the surgeon and the assistant to work seated, which is much less tiring. With this in view the position and height of the table and chair, instrument trolleys and other apparatus are adjusted before the operation is commenced. In the dental surgery this should be done before the surgeon and his assistant scrub up.

The mouth can be held open with a rubber prop placed between the molar teeth. For operations under local anaesthesia a prop so used often helps the patient by resting his muscles and joints. Under general anaesthesia the mouth must not be opened by force because of the danger of fracturing teeth or damaging the temporomandibular joint. Pressure intraorally on the mental protuberance will open the mouth or gags may be gently applied to the teeth to separate the jaws.

Before starting the operation the surgeon must make sure he has the right patient and notes. He then examines the mouth and radiographs to confirm the proposed operation. Where the patient is given a general anaesthetic teeth can be damaged or dislodged during induction. Especial care must be taken by anaesthetists and surgeons where loose teeth are present.

The close of the operation

The surgeon refers to the notes to confirm that all the surgery planned has been completed and tells the anaesthetist he is about to finish. He makes certain that all bleeding is controlled and that wound closure is satisfactory. He checks that packs or drains to be left in the mouth or wound are securely sutured in place. The mouth is searched for any clot, debris or swabs and a count is made of the teeth extracted, of swabs, needles and small instruments. With the anaesthetist's agreement the end of the throat pack may be drawn forward and any debris in the superficial layers removed from the mouth, after which the patient is handed over to the anaesthetist.

The surgeon will then write up the notes of the operation. This is done immediately for the information of the ward sister and whosoever should be called in an emergency.

Operation notes may be written in the following form:

Date	Name and number of theatre or surgery	Time of commencement of operation
	Surgeon named	
	Anaesthetist named	

1. Anaesthetic. Local anaesthetic, general anaesthetic, type, pack used.

2. Operation described logically. Incision – reflection – bone removed – teeth extracted or fracture reduced and fixed, etc. debridement of wound – closure of wound – sutures – dressings applied – removal of throat pack – condition of patient on finishing – time of completion of operation.

The assistant will remain with the anaesthetist to man the suction apparatus and to advise about the operation site. The patient must remain under the supervision of the anaesthetist preferably in a special recovery area, until he is sufficiently recovered to control his own airway.

It is usual in hospital practice for a nurse from the ward to fetch the patient from the operating theatre. The anaesthetist and the surgeon should tell her what procedures have taken place and give instructions verbally and in writing for the immediate post-operative nursing. She should be shown the site of the operation, the tongue suture if used, and any areas to be protected from pressure. Where intermaxillary fixation with wires or elastics is in place the nurse in shown which to cut to release the jaw in an emergency and given wire cutters for this purpose.

The patient will travel on a trolley equipped with an oxygen cylinder and mask, a tray containing tongue forceps, a gag and swabs firmly held in forceps. He will lie on his side in the recovery position (Fig. 4.4) to allow saliva or blood to drain from his mouth and will be accompanied back to the ward by two persons. One of these should be a trained nurse who gives the patient her undivided attention and in an emergency can send her companion for assistance.

Further reading

Cottone, J.A., Terezhalmy, G.T. & Molinari, J.A. (1995) *Practical Infection Control in Dentistry*, 2nd edn. Williams and Wilkins Media, Philadelphia.

Mulcahy, L., Rosenthal, M.M. & Lloyd-Bostock, S.M. (1998) *Medical Mishaps: pieces of the puzzle*. Open University Press, Buckingham.

Sentinel events: approaches to error reduction and prevention (1998). *Joint Commission Journal on Quality Improvement*. **24**(4), 175–86.

Chapter 7
Surgical Principles and Technique

Principles of:
- Painless surgery
- Asepsis
- Minimal damage
- Adequate access
- Arrest of haemorrhage
- Debridement
- Drainage
- Repair of wounds
- Control and prevention of infection of wounds
- Support of patient

The practice of surgery rests on certain fundamental principles which remain unchanged, though to apply them the surgeon may have to modify his technique to suit the anatomical field, the type of operation and the conditions obtaining at the time. The surgeon must have a clear and comprehensive knowledge of surgical physiology, of the anatomy of the region he is operating, and of the pathology of the condition under treatment.

Principle of painless surgery

Today it is accepted that all surgery should be painless. This is important to avoid psychological and physical stress to the patient which may predispose to shock, delay recovery and make surgery under local anaesthesia more difficult for the surgeon. In oral surgery it is wise for general anaesthetics to be administered by a specialist in this field, whereas the dental surgeon is usually highly skilled in giving his own local anaesthetic injections.

It is outside the scope of this book to discuss the administration of local and general anaesthetics. The choice between these will depend on surgical as well as medical considerations, and where doubt exists the decision should be made jointly with the anaesthetist. The dental surgeon may often have to guide the patient and the anaesthetist as to which is better.

The indications for general anaesthesia are: first, when there is an acute or subacute infection which it is not possible to treat using regional block anaesthesia; second, where the operation involves several quadrants of the mouth, is lengthy, difficult or of an alarming nature; third, for young children and adult patients who are unable to co-operate. General anaesthetics without intubation should not be used for procedures expected to last more than 5 minutes although use of a laryngeal mask can prolong this safely up to 20 minutes. As an out-patients procedure this is now almost entirely restricted for the treatment of children. Day-case surgery, where the patient is intubated and the post-operative period supervised by the nursing staff, is suitable for operations which can be completed within 45 minutes.

Local anaesthesia is suitable for many minor oral surgical procedures. It is indicated where the patient has eaten recently and does not wish to wait and in certain medical conditions (such as chronic bronchitis). The combination of local anaesthesia and sedation with intravenous benzodiazepines, such as midazolam, is useful for the nervous patient. This technique requires well trained staff and adequate recovery facilities. It should be treated in a similar fashion to a general anaesthetic and the patients prepared in the same way.

Principle of asepsis

Asepsis is the exclusion of micro-organisms from the operative field to prevent them entering the wound. The patient's mouth, however, cannot be sterilised and remains a source of infection. A pre-operative scaling and good oral hygiene practised before operation will reduce the chance of gross contamination; moreover patients seem to acquire a degree of immunity to their own oral flora.

The sterile instruments, fluids and dressings used in oral surgery are laid up on a trolley. Where pre-packed instruments are not used this must be done with sterile forceps. The surgeon and assistant should wear sterile disposable gloves and only those instruments laid on the trolley should be handled. A third person should be present to adjust the operating lights and position of the patient.

Principle of minimal damage

Inexperienced surgeons often pay too much attention to the tooth, cyst or tumour to be removed and too little to the tissues left after surgery is complete. Certain radical operations may regrettably require the sacrifice of vital structures but this does not often apply in oral surgery, and damage or loss of function as a result of carelessness or lack of foresight is inexcusable.

The commonest causes of trauma are poorly planned operations with ill-designed flaps, a careless approach to bone removal and tooth extraction, and excessive use of force by the surgeon or his assistant in dissection, retraction of flaps and in the use of elevators, burs and chisels. These practices increase postoperative pain and swelling and delay healing. They not only interfere with healing but increase the possibility of infection because they leave behind pieces of dead bone, tooth and mutilated soft tissues.

Principle of adequate access

Incision and flap

Access to the site of operation is gained by cutting the skin or mucous membrane and by dissecting through this incision to lay back a flap. The site, size and form of the incision is planned to give the best possible approach with the least danger to important nearby structures. The operation completed, the flap has a second and equally important function, that of providing the first dressing to the wound. To do this it must be large enough to give easy access, be mobilised with sufficient subcutaneous tissue to give adequate support and bring with it a good blood supply. It should have healthy, clean edges which will heal by first intention. This means that, in the mouth, when the mucoperiosteum is reflected the mucosa and periosteum must not be separated. The incision must be so designed that it does not cut across the blood supply to the flap but includes the vessels that supply that area of skin or mucous membrane, otherwise the edges may slough and healing is delayed (Fig. 7.1).

Where it covers a cavity in bone, it should be of such a size that when replaced the line of the incision rests securely on bone.

Incision

The scalpel is held in a pen-grip and the hand is supported against slipping. The incision is made with one firm, slow stroke of a sharp blade which is kept vertical to the epithelial surface. The bow is used for cutting, the point being kept above the skin or mucous membrane as a guide to the depth at which the incision is being made. (Fig. 7.2).

The point is used at the beginning and end of the incision to ensure an even depth of cut along the whole length. Mucoperiosteum should be cut through its full thickness down on to bone at *one* stroke.

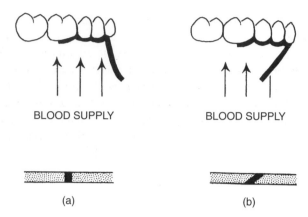

Fig. 7.1 (a) Above: Correct design of the buccal flap to ensure a satisfactory blood supply to all parts. Below: Cross-section of satisfactory incision made with the scalpel blade vertical to the surface of the skin. (b) Above: Incorrect design of buccal flap. Below: Cross-section of an incision made with the scalpel blade held obliquely.

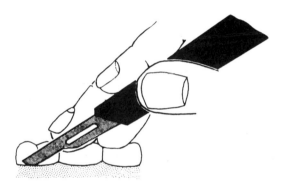

Fig. 7.2 The scalpel held in the pen-grip and the bow of no. 15 blade used to make the incision. Note the fingers supported on the teeth.

Dissection

The mucoperiosteal flap should be reflected with a periosteal elevator. A Howarth's raspatory may be used in this way, alternatively a Mitchells trimmer or an Ash or a Ward's periosteal elevator may be used. Holding an instrument in both hands to both retract and elevate using a 'knife and fork' technique can be useful. The instrument is first inserted into the incision and, starting in the buccal sulcus where the periosteum is loosely attached, the first few millimetres at the edge of the flap are gently freed along its periphery. Thereafter, it is reflected evenly along its whole length by a clean movement, with the end of the Howarth's raspatory pressed and kept firmly against the bone. Lifting movements are to be avoided as they tend to tear the tissues.

A skin flap is raised by separating it, with sufficient supporting tissue, from the underlying structures either by blunt dissection, using scissors, or, where necessary, by cutting with a scalpel. The essential point is to maintain an even depth of supporting tissue with an adequate blood supply and to avoid 'buttonholing' the flap. The deeper tissues are explored by blunt dissection with either sinus forceps, the fingers, or where delicate structures are involved by separating each layer by gently packing wet gauze between them. Connective tissue, muscle and bone must be identified, laid open in turn, and all important structures carefully preserved.

Cutting of bone

In oral surgery the cutting of bone to give access is done with burs, the efficiency of modern dental handpieces and sharp burs giving superlative control. However, chisels, gouges, rongeurs and files may also be used on occasion.

Burs

Tungsten carbide burs of medium size, either rosehead (Ash 7-16) or fissure (Ash 7-12), are used. Satisfactory cutting with fine control can only be attained using high speeds and minimal pressure. To avoid overheating of the tissues and clogging of the bur this must be irrigated with sterile saline.

Burs can be used in two ways, either to grind bone away or to remove blocks of bone. Grinding is done with rosehead or fissure burs preferably used with a gentle sweeping movement over the whole length of the area concerned, thereby leaving a smooth even edge. Blocks of bone are removed using fissure burs (Ash size 7) to make cuts through the cortex into the medulla round an area which can then be prised out.

Chisels

These may be used in young patients, under 40 years of age, where the natural lines of cleavage along the 'grain' of the bone are present. In the mandible these run vertically in the ascending ramus (almost parallel to the posterior border) and horizontally in the body (parallel to the occlusal surface). In the maxilla there is no true grain, but the thin plates of bone are easily cut. In older patients (over 40 years) the use of chisels is contraindicated as the bone is brittle and the mandible may shatter in unpredictable planes. Chisels may be used either by hand or more usually with a mallet. In either case they must be supported firmly against slipping. Some resilience should be provided in the mallet either in the handle or by use of a soft head.

The chisel may be used to plane bone away or to cut out blocks of bone. The direction in which the chisel cuts is determined by the angle of the bevelled surface. When used as a plane the bevelled face is placed against the bone and driven along at the required depth to shave off successive wafers. To remove blocks of bone the bevelled surface is usually turned towards the bone which is to be left).

Chisels and burs

These may be combined by using a rosehead bur (No. 7) to drill holes to the required depth at intervals of 3–5 mm along the planned line of the cut. The holes are then joined with a chisel and the cut deepened gradually till the bone splits off. This method is especially useful for removing large pieces of bone safely.

Rongeurs and files

These instruments are used mostly for trimming and smoothing bone edges when the operation has been completed. The rongeurs may also be used for cutting alveolar bone in alveolectomy and thin plates of bone such as those covering dental cysts.

Retraction

Retraction has two objects, to provide free access for the surgeon and to protect the tissues. It is the most important task undertaken by the assistant, which, if badly performed, can be a positive hindrance. The tissue layers divided by the incision and the dissection are gently held back with instruments (Fig. 7.3). There should be no tugging or rough handling, for if this is necessary the incision is too small and needs to be enlarged. Retractors must not be moved without warning as they may accidentally obscure the field or deflect an instrument. To keep still for periods, without tiring, the hands must be in a comfortable position, if possible supported in some way. Thus the blade of the retractor under a mucoperiosteal flap should rest against the alveolar bone. The surgeon should pause at intervals to allow his assistant to rest and readjust his position.

Damage may also occur from compressing or cutting the lips or cheeks against the teeth. To avoid undue pressure at any one point, the lips, tongue and cheeks are best held back by broad-bladed instruments (Fig. 7.4). Unfortunately, this is more often done by the handles of retractors, the blades of which are holding back flaps in the mouth and only a few of which are designed for both purposes. Sutures of thick silk can be passed through all these structures, and through mucoperiosteal flaps, to hold them (Fig. 7.4).

Cleansing the field of operation

The assistant cleanses the field of operation of fluids and loose debris, which might obscure the surgeon's view or remain in the wound to become foreign bodies. Large fragments should be lifted out with fine forceps as soon as they

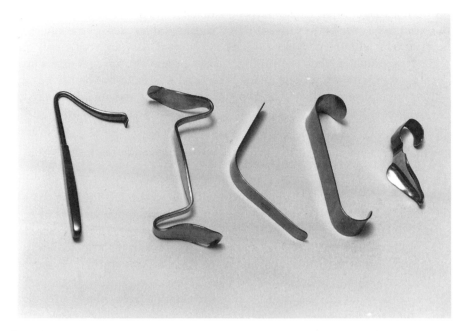

Fig. 7.3   Retractors. Left to right: Bowdler-Henry rake retractor, Ward's double ended third molar retractor, Lack's tongue depressor, Kilner's cheek retractor, Laster's retractor for upper third molars.

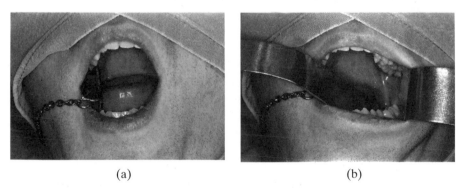

(a)   (b)

Fig. 7.4   (a) Mouth prop in position between teeth with safety chain; (b) Lack's tongue depressor and Kilner's cheek retractor in position to allow access to left side of the mouth.

are seen, otherwise they may be lost. Blood, water and the minute debris from cutting hard tissues with the dental bur can be removed by suction. The tip of the sucker should be kept in one position, preferably at the point of dependent drainage, as moving it continually can interfere with the surgeon's instrumentation and, if rapid, causes a visual kaleidoscope effect. At intervals sterile water must be aspirated to prevent blood clotting in the tubing or connections. Large particles of bone or tags of tissue are avoided; they are sometimes musical but will eventually block the tubing. As this occurs not infrequently, a spare 'head' together with a stilette is needed. The sucker should not be used as a retractor or to explore wounds or sockets as it can cause damage and may encourage bleeding. The use of swabs in similar circumstances avoids this.

Principle of arrest of haemorrhage

The natural arrest of haemorrhage and the pathological conditions which may lead to abnormal bleeding together with their management have been discussed in Chapter 3. At operation the arrest of primary haemorrhage depends on the application of pressure to the vessel walls, which to be effective must be maintained for at least the time taken for the blood to clot. Haemostatis must be achieved in each quadrant of the mouth before continuing to other procedures in a new area. Reactionary and secondary haemorrhage are discussed in Chapter 10.

Soft tissues

Digital pressure
This is particularly useful for capillary or venous bleeding and as an immediate measure when a large vessel has been cut. It is applied either by compressing the tissues, or the offending vessel, against bone or in certain situations, such as the lip, by exerting pressure between index finger and thumb. The lingual artery may be controlled by drawing the tongue forward so that the artery is pressed against the hyoid bone. The facial artery crosses the lower border of the mandible where digital pressure may be applied.

Haemostats or artery forceps
Where a vessel is cut during operation it must be found swiftly and secured with artery forceps. For small vessels the haemostats may be removed after twisting two or three times, but on larger vessels they must be replaced by ligatures.

Ligatures
Direct ligature of a vessel is performed preferably before division. Artery forceps are placed above and below where the cut is to be made and after division resorbable ligatures are firmly tied and the haemostats removed (Fig. 7.5).

In major haemorrhage from the jaws not controlled by local measures it is on occasion necessary to ligate the external carotid artery. The collateral blood

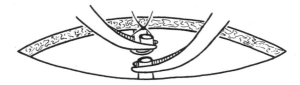

Fig. 7.5 Use of haemostats. Note the position of the lower haemostats on the vessel so that after division the beaks curve upwards out of the wound (as on the upper haemostats) to facilitate passing and tying of the ligature.

supply and anastomosis is so good in the face that it is often necessary to do this on both sides, if it is to be effective. A sufficient blood supply is still maintained by the other lesser vessels serving this area.

Packing

As a temporary measure ribbon gauze soaked in saline may be packed into operative or traumatic wounds and held under pressure for a short interval to arrest haemorrhage. Oxidised cellulose wound packs are useful to obtain haemostasis and may be left in the wounds as they are bioresorbable.

Posture

The position of the patient both during and after operation may help to reduce the blood pressure in the bleeding part. In dental haemorrhage the patient is kept sitting upright or propped up with pillows in bed unless shocked or fainting.

Electrocoagulation

This may be applied directly to the vessels or by passing the current through the artery forceps clamping the vessels. Monopolar diathermy uses an adhesive pad on the patient to complete the electrical circuit, whereas in bipolar diathermy current passes between the beaks of the specially insulated forceps.

Bleeding from bone

Capillary oozing from bone surfaces may be controlled by burnishing the bone with a small instrument or by applying for a few minutes hot packs prepared by soaking gauze squares in very hot water and wringing out the excess. Bone wax rubbed into the surface of the bone is also very effective in occluding small vessels, but should be removed prior to closure as it can cause foreign body reactions.

Where an artery is bleeding from a bone surface it may be compressed by driving a chisel into the bone near to it and forcing a wedge of bone against the vessel.

Principle of debridement (toilet of wounds)

The operation completed, the wound is prepared for closure by careful cleansing to remove debris, a major cause of post-operative infection. Pathological tissue, such as tooth follicle or sinus tracts, is excised. The bone cavity is saucerised where necessary, and the edges filed to a clean smooth finish without sharp projections. The flaps are trimmed of all necrotic tissue or tags. Tooth chips and loose pieces of bone, not attached to periosteum, are removed from the wound which is then thoroughly irrigated with saline.

Principle of drainage

Wounds need to drain freely after operation where they are contaminated or infected, where an abscess has been incised, or where immediate closure is made over a dead space which may fill with blood or serum and subsequently become infected.

Fine superficial drains

These are made of pieces of rubber glove and are used in wounds of the face to allow escape of tissue exudate. They are usually removed after 48 hours (Fig. 7.6a).

Larger superficial drains

Corrugated rubber or a Yeates drain is used in a dental abscess to keep the wound edges apart and allow thick pus to flow freely (Fig. 7.6b). Though chiefly used for extraoral incisions and drainage they are necessary for large collections of pus drained intraorally.

Deep drains

Tubing, sometimes with small holes cut in its walls, is used in osteomyelitis of the jaws or to drain the antrum through the nose. The tubes must be of sufficient diameter to ensure the free passage of fluid and to allow irrigation with saline or antibiotic solutions.

Vacuum drains

These are inserted at a point remote from the wound by means of a central sharp stylet. The stylet is then withdrawn leaving the tube drain in position. The latter is attached to a plastic bottle from which the air has been expressed. The advantages of vacuum drains are that they are inserted away from the operation wound and the negative pressure developed assists removal of fluid (Fig. 7.6c).

Drains should be inserted into a cavity at its most dependent point and they must be fixed by a suture or some other device to prevent them falling out of, or being drawn into, the wound. They should be examined daily to ensure that

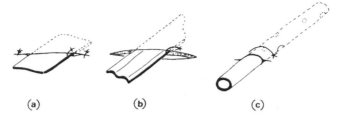

Fig. 7.6   Drains: (a) Rubber glove drain; (b) Corrugated rubber drain; (c) Suction drains attached to vacuum bottles. An airtight seal must be achieved around the exit site of the drain by careful suturing.

they are patent and serving their function. They are removed when the discharge has ceased, usually between the third and seventh day. Long drains may be shortened before this, particularly when they are near major vessels which they may erode.

An entry must be made in the patient's records both when they are put in and when they are removed.

Principle of repair of wounds

Before commencing closure the surgeon makes sure that the operation has been satisfactorily completed, that bleeding is arrested and that all swabs, instruments and teeth are accounted for. Closure is carried out by suturing the wound for which purpose many forms of needle holder, needle and suture material are available.

Needle holder

The Kilner needle holder is commonly used in the mouth. The ratcheted handles provide a firm grip of the needle (Fig. 7.7).

Needles

These may be round or triangular in cross-section; the latter are called 'cutting needles'. They may be of various shapes but the half-round or curved needle is used on the mucous membranes and skin of the face. The size of the needle should be such that it can be passed through the flap without ever holding it by either the tail or the point, where it may easily be broken.

Suture materials

Silk is the most economical and is to be preferred in the mouth if wound support is required for a precise period; however, resorbable sutures are most frequently used in the mouth. Catgut may only give wound support for a few days whilst

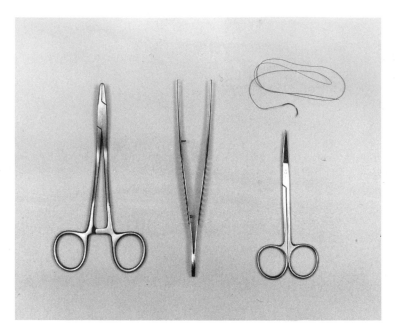

Fig. 7.7 Suture kit. Left to right: Kilner's needle holder, Gillies toothed tissue forceps, suture scissors, and above, suture.

Vicryl^R may last for several weeks. Resorbable sutures have the advantage of not requiring removal and thus allay patient anxiety. Fine (5/0 or 6/0) nylon monofilament sutures are used for facial wounds. Staples can be used for rapid closure of neck or scalp wounds but should not be used on the face.

Suturing

To suture the mucoperiosteum the edges of the wound are apposed to confirm that closure can be made without tension. Where one side is fixed to bone the first 3 mm of the margin are freed to make the passage of the needle easy. The flap is picked up and held everted with toothed tissue forceps applied at right angles to the free edge of the flap (Fig. 7.8). A curved cutting needle (22 mm) with silk (3/0) is passed through from the outer surface of the mucoperiosteum close to the tissue forceps which splint the flap against the pressure from the needle. The suture must go through the periosteum and should be placed about 3 mm from the free edge to prevent it pulling out when tied. The other side is similarly everted and the needle passed through from the raw surface with an equal bite. To make sure that the final position will be satisfactory the margins of the wound are drawn together with the suture before it is tied with a surgeon's knot (Fig. 7.9). It should not be tied too tightly as this may cause the edges to overlap and because subsequent swelling may cause ischaemia at the wound margins. Sufficient sutures are inserted to prevent the wound gaping at any point.

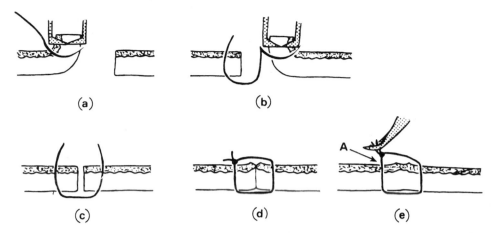

Fig. 7.8 (a), (b) and (c) show eversion of the flap and the needle passed obliquely through the tissue; (d) tying of the suture everts the edges of the wound; (e) removal of sutures, by cutting at A and thereby avoiding drawing the exposed part of the suture through the tissues.

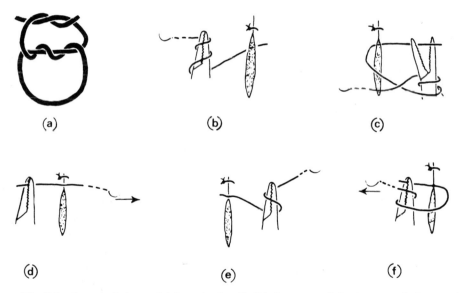

Fig. 7.9 Surgeon's knot: (a) knot in detail; (b) first part of the knot made by passing suture round needle holder; (c) and (d) short free end grasped and knot slid off beaks; (e) and (f) second part of knot made by passing suture round the needle holder in the opposite direction.

Skin incisions are closed in layers, the fascial and muscle planes being identified and re-apposed. They are sutured with catgut or polyglycolic acid, the knot of which should be tied inwards and the free ends cut very short to avoid irritation. The deep sutures should take all the necessary strain so that the skin lies in correct apposition and may be stitched without tension, which is a cause of scarring. It is very important that the skin margins are held everted with the raw surfaces in apposition to ensure rapid healing (Fig. 7.8).

Types of suture

Simple interrupted sutures

Simple interrupted sutures are of almost universal application. They are inserted singly through each side of the wound and tied with a surgeon's knot (Fig. 7.9). Several of these may be used at short intervals between 4 and 8 mm apart to close large wounds, so that the tension is shared and therefore not high at any one point (Fig. 7.10a). When put in correctly they will evert the edges of the flap. Should one break or pull out only this one need be replaced. The wound is free of interference between each stitch and is easy to keep clean.

Horizontal mattress suture

A horizontal mattress suture has the property of everting the mucosal or skin margins, thereby bringing greater areas of raw tissue into contact. For this reason it is useful for closing wounds over bony deficiencies such as oro-antral fistulae or cyst cavities (Fig. 7.10b).

Vertical mattress sutures

Specially designed for use in the skin, vertical mattress sutures pass through it at two levels, one deep to provide support and adduction of the wound surface at a depth and one superficial to draw the edges together and evert them.

Continuous sutures

Continuous sutures all suffer from the great disadvantage that if they cut out at one point the suture slackens along the whole length of the wound which will then gape open. They have the advantage in the mouth that only two knots with their associated tags are present. The simple continuous suture (Fig. 7.10c), though easy to insert, applies its pull on the wound in an oblique direction. The continuous blanket stitch suture is far more stable and firm and gives traction on the wound edges at right angles to the wound (Fig. 7.10d). The purse-string suture is useful as a deep suture for wounds of the skin of the face, but care must be taken that in drawing the suture taut there is no wrinkling or creasing of the skin edges.

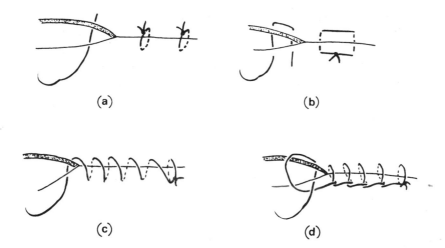

Fig. 7.10 Sutures: (a) simple interrupted; (b) horizontal mattress; (c) simple continuous; (d) continuous blanket stitch.

Knots

The knots used to tie sutures are the reef-knot and surgeon's knot. They may be tied with the fingers but this is difficult to do in the mouth and it is important to master the technique of tying them with the needle holder as illustrated (Fig. 7.9). The knot when tied must lie well on one side of the line of the wound.

Removal of sutures

Sutures in mucous membrane are removed after 5 to 7 days. In the skin alternate stitches are often taken out about the third to fifth day and the remainder between the fifth and eighth days. A good guide is that as soon as they begin to get loose they should be taken out. They should first be cleaned and then removed as shown in Fig. 7.8.

Principle of control and prevention of infection of wounds

The incidence of post-operative infection will be reduced by careful pre-operative preparation, an aseptic technique, minimal trauma and adequate drainage. Post-operatively the tissues may be protected by the use of dressings.

In the mouth surgical incisions are not dressed except where there is a deficiency of mucous membrane over bone, when packs are used to cover it. Small skin incisions are normally dressed with dry gauze, until the formation of serous exudate has stopped when they are best left uncovered. More extensive wounds and abrasions may be covered with tulle-gras and dry gauze strapped into position with adhesive surgical tape. Where a drain is *in situ*, gauze is placed round it for support, and to absorb the discharge cotton wool is held over it by a bandage or strapping which should completely cover the dressing.

Packs are used to protect exposed bone or to prevent skin or mucous membrane from closing over a wound which should heal from its base by granulation. They can in no way serve as drains. Ribbon gauze impregnated with BIPP or Whitehead's varnish is packed firmly but not tightly into the cavity. When inserted under a general anaesthetic, packs must be sutured into place lest they come loose and obstruct the airway. They should not be changed too frequently and *both insertion and removal must be entered in the patient's notes.*

Antibacterial therapy

Views on the prophylactic use of antibiotics vary but on no account should they take the place of an aseptic technique. In oral surgery it is impossible to obtain a sterile field and many patients present with acute or chronic inflammatory conditions such as advanced periodontal disease, pericoronitis or contaminated fractures. For this reason many oral surgeons prefer to operate under an antibiotic cover, but it should not be prescribed routinely. Each case must be assessed individually and bacterial culture and antibiotic sensitivity tests obtained wherever possible. The prescription of antibacterial drugs is discussed in Chapter 5.

Principle of support of the patient

The pre- and post-operative care and the general support of the patient have been discussed in Chapter 2.

Further reading

Taylor, I. & Karran, S.J. (1996) *Surgical Principles*. Arnold, London.

Chapter 8
Extraction of Teeth and Roots

- Examination and assessment
- Extraction of teeth
- Elevators
- Extraction procedure
- Extractions in children
- Fracture of tooth
- Transveolar approach
- Removal of roots
- Arrest of haemorrhage
- Post-extraction instructions

Indications for extraction:

- Caries
- Periodontal disease
- Trauma
- Orthodontics
- Involvement in pathology
  - infection
  - cysts
  - tumours

Examination and assessment

A full medical history is necessary before attempting extractions as these are contraindicated in certain conditions such as leukaemias and for patients whose jaws have undergone irradiation. Other medical conditions which need special preparation, such as bone dysplasias and cardiac and haemorrhagic diseases, are discussed in Chapter 3. Any previous difficulty with extractions, including post-operative bleeding or infection, is noted and if serious in extent investigated further.

Clinical examination

The patient's sex, age, general build and bone structure are significant. Heavily built men, have teeth difficult to extract whilst in old age roots are brittle and the bone sclerosed, the so-called 'glass in concrete syndrome'. Access may be difficult in children who have small mouths and in patients with facial scars or trismus.

The tooth to be extracted is examined. Teeth misplaced palatally or lingually, rotated, inclined, or single standing teeth in occlusion, are all potentially difficult. Certain teeth frequently have abnormal root formation, particularly the upper and lower third molars. Heavily filled and dead teeth or those suffering from long-standing periodontal disease tend to become brittle. Periodontal disease predisposes to post-operative bleeding and infection. In acute ulcerative gingivitis or where the gingival condition suggests a blood dyscrasia, all extractions must be delayed until these have been treated.

Radiographic examination

The nature of the root form and bone structure can only be determined from radiographs, and ideally these should always be taken before extraction, but in practice this is done when the history or examination suggests the extractions will be difficult. It should be a routine procedure for all lower third molars and misplaced teeth. Intraoral periapical views should show the whole of the crown, root and alveolus and demonstrate the relationship of the roots to such important structures as the maxillary sinus and the inferior dental canal. Radiographs must be examined carefully as certain features, such as extra roots on molar teeth, are easily missed.

Assessment

All the findings on examination and radiography are considered, particularly the number, size, shape and position of roots and any signs of hypercementosis or resorption. The condition of the supporting bone, especially evidence of sclerosis, resorption or of secondary conditions such as apical granulomas and cysts, is noted. Where any of these complications occur the treatment plan should be modified to meet them.

Extraction of teeth

Extraction of teeth:

- Knowledge of tooth morphology
- Application of force related to tooth morphology
- Use of forceps
- Use of elevators to assist and facilitate
- Position of patient vital to success

Tooth morphology

For the surgeon to extract teeth successfully it is important to understand the morphology of the roots of the tooth which is to be extracted. Only then can force be applied appropriately to remove the tooth.

Upper incisors and canines

Upper incisors and canines have single, conical roots and are therefore rotated with a purposeful action, the forceps turning through as wide an arc as possible without damaging adjacent teeth (Fig. 8.3). The upper canine, because its root is slightly flattened mesiodistally, can be extracted by an outward buccal movement if it is resistant to rotation.

Upper premolars

Upper premolars have either one strong root markedly flattened mediodistally or two fine conical roots placed buccally and palatally. They are extracted by a limited bucco-palatal movement lest the apices should break.

Upper first and second molars

Upper first and second molars both have three roots which are usually somewhat flattened. The palatal diverges strongly from the two buccal roots. They are taken buccally with a long, steady movement whilst the upward pressure is maintained (Fig. 8.3). Palatal movement is contraindicated as it may cause the palatal root to fracture.

Upper third molars

The morphology of upper third molar roots varies widely; some are fused, others have three fine roots. They are extracted in the same way as the other upper molars, but it is wise to take a radiograph first.

Lower incisors and canines

The roots of lower incisors and canines are flattened mesiodistally and as the buccal plate of bone is very weak they are extracted with an outward buccal movement.

Lower premolars

Lower premolars and canines have conical roots and are therefore rotated.

Lower first and second molars

The roots of lower first and second molars are flattened mesiodistally. They should be extracted by a buccal movement while the downward pressure is maintained.

Lower third molars

A wide variation occurs in the root form of lower third molars and in their position in the mandible as they are often misplaced or inclined. Radiographs should always be taken before extraction which may require an open or transalveolar approach.

Deciduous teeth

The upper and lower incisors and canines are extracted with the same movements used for their permanent successors. The molar teeth, however, have divergent roots which enclose the follicle of the developing premolar teeth and it is possible to remove or damage the latter when extracting a deciduous molar. Great care must be taken in using the forceps, which should not be driven too far up the periodontal membrane. They are applied to the tooth *root*, avoiding the bifurcation under which the permanent tooth germ nestles.

Where, owing to caries or a fracture of the tooth during surgery, a deciduous molar root is retained which cannot be grasped with the forceps, it may be extracted by applying a right-angled Warwick James elevator to the mesial aspect of mesial roots or distal aspect of distal roots to elevate them gently along their natural curvature. Should there be a risk of damaging the underlying permanent tooth, then the retained root is best left and the patient's parent told the reason.

Forceps

Forceps are designed to apply appropriate forces to the teeth. They have two blades with sharp edges to cut the periodontal fibres. The blades are wedge-shaped to dilate the socket and are hollowed on their inner surface to fit the roots. They are made in various sizes and a range should be available so that a pair may be selected which fit snugly round the roots and have even contact with the cementum over a wide area. One- or two-point contact is bad and prevents the tooth being gripped firmly. They should engage only the roots and never the crowns of the teeth.

The blades are hinged which allows them to close and grasp the root. The handles act as a lever which gives the operator a mechanical advantage. The farther from the blades the surgeon grasps the handles the less effort he will have to make to apply force to the tooth. In order to drive the forceps blade straight up the long axis of the tooth the shape of the handle is varied. Lower forceps have handles at right angles to the blades, upper forceps are straight for anterior teeth and cranked for the posteriors. For the upper third molars the beaks as well as the handles are bent (Fig. 8.1).

Extraction of teeth with forceps

The extraction of teeth is a surgical operation based primarily on an anatomical appreciation of their attachment in the jaws. First the soft tissues of the gingival attachment and periodontal membrane are cut to separate the tooth

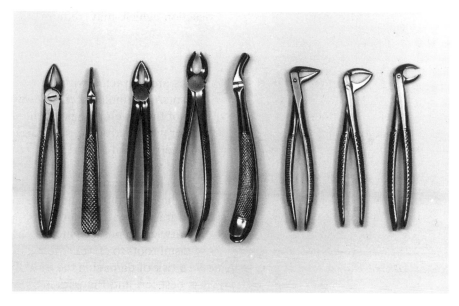

Fig. 8.1 Extraction forceps. Left to right: Upper straights, side view upper straights, upper premolars, upper molars, side view upper molars, lower straights, lower premolars, lower molars.

from bone. Next the socket is dilated either by instruments with wedge-shaped blades which are driven along the periodontal membrane, or by moving the root to expand its bony socket. Finally when the tooth is loose it may be drawn out of the alveolus. When completed with forceps, extractions are performed in two movements.

First movement

This is the same for all the teeth of both jaws. The forceps are applied on the buccal and the palatal or lingual aspect of the tooth, regardless of whether it is normally or abnormally positioned in the arch. For multirooted teeth, unless full forceps are used, the blades must be kept on a root, not the bifurcation. The blades are passed carefully under the gingival margin of the tooth avoiding damage to the soft tissues, and driven up or down the roots (according to the jaw concerned) in the same plane as the long axis of the tooth to penetrate as far as possible. This can only be done successfully if the forceps blades are held sufficiently apart that they do *not* grip the tooth root.

Considerable force is used, particularly in the upper jaw. In the lower jaw this must be limited to that which the operator can counteract by supporting the mandible with his free hand. Whilst driving up the root in this way the blades should be in contact with the root surface but not gripping it. This movement cuts the gingival attachment and periodontal membrane and also uses the

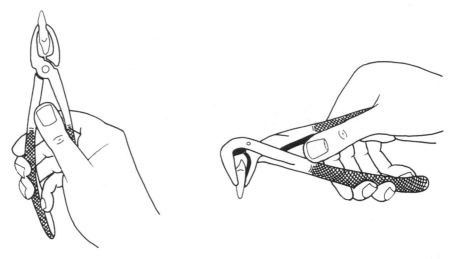

Fig. 8.2   Left: Method of holding upper forceps. Note grip and position of the blades on root, *not* crown. Right: Method of holding lower forceps.

wedge-shaped blades to dilate the socket. Conical roots may sometimes be extracted by this movement alone.

Second movement

The first movement completed, the blades of the forceps are closed to grasp the root and a second movement is performed which by moving the tooth roots uses them to dilate further the socket and to free them from the periodontal membrane. During this action, to prevent the blades slipping off the tooth, a firm vertical pressure up or down the long axis of the root must be maintained. The character of the second movement depends on two factors. Firstly, in both upper and lower jaws the palatal or lingual alveolar bone is thicker than the buccal bone, and secondly, the anatomy of the roots of the various classes of teeth differs both in their number and shape.

Considering the upper first molar in more detail it can be seen that two forces are applied to the tooth (Fig. 8.3). If a buccal force is applied alone this produces a rotation of the tooth which is likely to cause a fracture. If a greater upwards force is applied simultaneously this produces a rotation approximately through the apices of the buccal roots and this allows the whole of the buccal surface of the tooth to expand the socket. The palatal root is pulled out of the socket along its arc of curvature. This mechanical principle can be applied to lower molar teeth also.

The use of excess force is avoided, and every effort is made to develop 'feeling' through the forceps. This enables the surgeon to recognise resistance to excursions in certain directions and to exploit other movements which the tooth will follow more easily, and so to extract always along the line of least resistance.

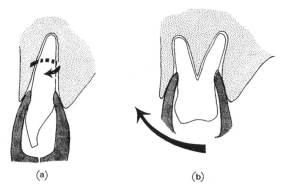

Fig. 8.3 Movements in the extraction of teeth: (a) rotation; (b) buccal outward movement.

Difficult extractions

The ultimate aim of the student is to acquire the ability to assess the tooth he wishes to extract and to modify his technique accordingly. During the operation the second movement is always slow, steady and purposeful and not a series of short, jerky, shaking gestures which are both ineffective and unpleasant for the patient.

Should there be complete resistance to the forceps when the usual pressure is applied the operation is stopped and a new assessment made with radiographs. Where necessary the roots are freed through a transalveolar approach by making a flap, removing bone and dividing the tooth, rather than by exerting more and more force till the tooth breaks.

Elevators

Elevators are single-bladed instruments for extracting teeth and roots, which they do by moving them out of the sockets along a path determined by the natural curvature of the roots. They are applied to the cementum on any surface, usually the mesial, distal or buccal, at a point (the point of application) where there is alveolar bone to provide them with a fulcrum. An adjoining tooth must never be used as the fulcrum, unless it is also to be extracted at the same visit, as it might be loosened accidentally.

Elevators are supported against slipping by resting the forefingers of the working hand on an adjacent tooth or the jaw (Fig. 8.4). They may be pushed firmly *between tooth and bone* to engage the point of application, but when elevating the tooth the force used is carefully controlled and should not exceed that which can be applied by rotating the instrument between finger and thumb (Fig. 8.5). Where this is insufficient to move the tooth, other measures such as removal of bone or division of the tooth may be necessary. An elevator should never be used as a class 1 lever, that is like a crowbar, as bone

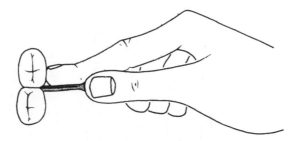

Fig. 8.4   Application of an elevator to a lower right molar tooth viewed from above. Note the palm grip and the index finger used as a support.

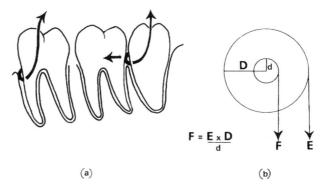

$$F = \frac{E \times D}{d}$$

(a)   (b)

Fig. 8.5   (a) Left: Correct point of application between tooth and bone. Right: Incorrect application between tooth and tooth. (b) The force applied at the elevator handle (E) is multiplied by the ratio of the diameter of the handle (D) to the diameter of the blade (d) at the point of application.

will be crushed and the mechanical advantage is such that the jaw may be fractured.

Throughout elevation its effects on the tooth to be extracted and on the adjacent teeth is carefully watched so that ineffective or damaging movements are avoided. Where a tooth is standing distal to the one to be extracted every precaution must be taken not to transmit injurious forces to it.

Many elevators have been designed to exert more than finger and thumb pressure, but these should not be used to extract teeth. A description follows of some elevators which are safe to use, provided the above principles are obeyed.

Coupland's elevator

Coupland's elevator is made in three sizes; each has a single blade not unlike that of the forceps (Fig. 8.6). It may be used as a wedge to dilate the socket when driven vertically up the periodontal membrane. More commonly it is used as a pulley lever, the mechanical advantage being obtained through the greater

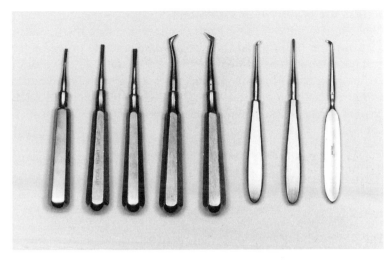

Fig. 8.6 Elevators. Left to right: Couplands 1, 2, and 3, Cryers left and right, Warwick James left, straight and right.

diameter of the handle over that of the blade (Fig. 8.5). When inserted horizontally between tooth and bone the sharp blade engages the point of application on the cementum and, with the alveolar bone as a fulcrum, the handle is rotated to lift the root out of its socket along its line of withdrawal (Figs. 8.4 and 8.5).

Warwick James elevators

Warwick James elevators are a pair of fine elevators (Fig. 8.6). The blade may be driven into the periodontal membrane to engage the root either mesially, distally or buccally and the handle rotated to lift it from its socket. A straight Warwick James elevator is also available and used in a similar way to the Coupland's elevator.

Cryer's elevators

Cryer's elevators are made in pairs, a right and left, and have a short, sharp-pointed, triangular blade at right angles to the handle (Fig. 8.6). They are used exactly like the right-angled Warwick James elevators but the larger, stronger blade gives them a superior mechanical advantage particularly when they are applied buccally to roots or to molar teeth at their bifurcation.

In molar teeth, especially in the mandible, where one root is retained a Cryer's elevator may be inserted into the adjacent empty socket and the sharp point used to remove the inter-radicular bone until it can engage the cementum. The bone is flaked away starting at the occlusal margin of the septum and working down towards the root apex.

The combined use of forceps and elevators

The combined use of these instruments will enable the operator to exploit the best qualities of both and thereby develop a gentle progressive technique. The first instrument to be applied should be a Coupland's elevator driven vertically up the long axis. This will cut the periodontal membrane and dilate the bony socket on both buccal and lingual aspects and indicate if undue resistance is present. As soon as there is some response to the elevators, forceps may be applied.

Extraction procedure

The supporting hand

The responsibility for seeing that the jaws are adequately supported rests with the operator, and his free hand is used for this purpose. This is particularly important in the mandible where the downward force must be resisted. Under local anaesthesia, a prop may be inserted and the patient can help by biting firmly on this. Under general anaesthesia the anaesthetist assists by supporting the mandible at the angles. Satisfactory support is equally important when using forceps or elevators (Fig. 8.7).

The other function of the supporting hand is to retract the cheeks and tongue and to protect the tissues. This is done by placing a finger and thumb (or two fingers) one on each side of the gum on the buccal and the lingual or palatal aspects of the tooth. At the same time the operator is able to feel that the blades of the forceps are indeed under the mucous membrane and correctly applied to the tooth. During the second movement of extraction, the watching fingers can feel any slipping of the forceps on the tooth or any tendency of adjacent teeth to move, or alveolar bone to fracture. When working on the maxilla the free fingers of the supporting hand should be kept closed to avoid the fingers causing accidental damage to the patient's eyes.

Stance

The right-handed operator stands facing the patient to the left of the chair but not too close as this makes lighting difficult. The stance has been compared to that of a boxer about to deliver a blow. The left foot is advanced, the weight balanced on both feet, with the arms slightly bent. The left hand is put forward to support the jaw whilst the right grasps the forceps. This position is adopted for the extraction of all upper teeth and for those in the left mandible (Fig. 8.8).

Teeth in the right mandible are extracted from behind the patient. The feet are apart with the right slightly advanced, and the left arm is placed round the patient's head to support the lower jaw (Figs. 8.7 and 8.8).

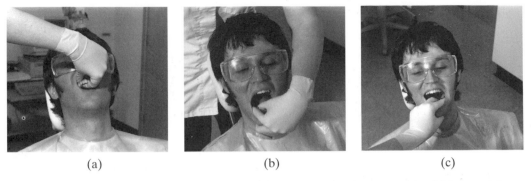

Fig. 8.7 Position of supporting hand: (a) for extraction in upper right; (b) lower right; (c) lower left. Note: finger and thumb used where possible to give sensitive feedback on tooth movement. Lower jaw must be adequately supported.

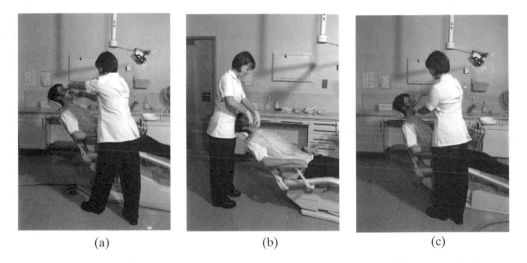

Fig. 8.8 Position of operator: (a) for extractions in upper jaw; (b) lower right; (c) lower left.

Chair position

The patient should be seated upright with the buttocks well back in the chair and the head supported with the neck slightly extended. The height of the chair is adjusted so that the operator has a clear view of the tooth without bending or twisting of the spine. A good posture should be maintained at all times. In general the chair is higher for extractions in the upper jaw and lower for those in the lower jaw.

Order of extraction of teeth

To prevent blood from the sockets of extracted teeth obscuring the field of operation it is usual to remove lower teeth before uppers, and posteriors before anteriors. Unnecessary movement to and fro about the chair is avoided by starting multiple extractions with those from the right mandible, which are the only ones done from behind on the sitting patient.

It is wise to begin with the most painful tooth when undertaking multiple extractions lest any surgical or anaesthetic difficulty prevents the completion of the operation. Similarly, when working under local anaesthesia only one quadrant of the mouth should be injected at a time. When the surgery in this area has been successfully completed a new quadrant may be injected. It is better to take out teeth from one side of the mouth only at one visit, thereby leaving the other comfortable for chewing.

The extraction of a great many teeth at one out-patient sitting is contraindicated as it may upset the patient and the blood loss can be considerable. It is not possible to state a figure for the number of teeth as much will depend on the surgical difficulty and the patient's health and morale, but between four and eight would seem reasonable. Where it is necessary to do more at one visit the patient should be kept in the recovery room for at least half an hour postoperatively and then accompanied home by a relative. Alternatively the patient should be admitted to hospital.

Extractions in children under out-patient general anaesthesia

The pre-operative preparation for general anaesthesia is discussed in Chapter 2.

Out-patient general anaesthetics are now restricted to facilities that are in close proximity to critical care and are reserved for children under 16. Use of sedation in the form of relative analgesia is becoming more common. Adults requiring a general anaesthetic are listed as day-cases, or if necessary as an in-patient.

The surgeon checks the patient's name, the teeth to be extracted, and that there are no loose teeth in the mouth. The patient is treated in the supine position. With the anaesthetist's agreement a prop, the smallest which will keep the mouth open widely, should be placed as far back in the mouth as possible. The prop must be inspected before it is put in place to ensure it is in good condition and that there is a chain firmly attached to it which can be left hanging out of the mouth (Fig. 7.4).

When induction is complete the mouth must always be packed with a length of gauze. The pack is inserted into the lingual sulcus to lift the tongue against the soft palate and thus occlude the oral airway. This should safeguard the nasal airway which the anaesthetist uses to maintain the anaesthetic. Care must be taken not to overpack. Whilst the teeth are being extracted the surgeon must not obstruct the airway, particularly by failing to support the lower jaw. He should beware when extracting from the upper jaw of damaging the lower lip by trapping it between forceps and lower teeth. All broken tooth fragments are removed from the mouth immediately, and, together with the extracted teeth, are placed in a special receptacle, care being taken not to carry them back into the mouth by accident.

On finishing the operation the prop and pack are removed by the person who put them in place, and the patient is turned on his side with the lower jaw held forward to allow blood to drain out of the mouth. The mandible is pushed into occlusion to check that the condyles are not dislocated (Chapter 17). The teeth are counted and all apices checked.

Extractions with the surgeon seated

The chair is adjusted with the patient supine and the surgeon seated on a mobile chair capable of moving in an arc about the patient's head (Fig. 8.9). Only one pattern of lower right-angled premolar forceps is necessary for all extractions in both upper and lower jaws. This is made possible by the use of both hands.

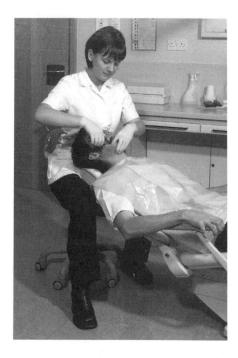

Fig. 8.9 Extractions with operator seated. Note: chair should be adjusted to allow a stable spine position.

The extractions are performed using the principles described previously in this chapter. The upper and lower teeth on the right side are extracted with the right hand, those on the patient's left with the left hand. Some slight modification of the supporting hand is necessary when working on the upper jaw, but the use of right-angled forceps does not require any change in the basic movements used in either jaw.

It must be emphasised that there are hazards in operating on a supine patient as displaced teeth, roots or fillings may fall back into the pharynx and the dental surgeon must take adequate steps to prevent this by getting the conscious patient to co-operate by turning his head well to one side during the operation. Further the assistant should have high power suction and a suitable instrument immediately available for grasping any displaced object. Under general anaesthesia the throat must be adequately packed off.

Fracture of the tooth

Fracture of the tooth during extraction occurs frequently, though its incidence may be reduced by a conscientious assessment and a careful progressive technique. Where the fracture is at or above the level of the margin of the alveolar bone and is thought to be due to brittleness or caries and not to excessive resistance, then the extraction may be continued using forceps and elevators as for standing teeth.

In other cases if the fracture is below the level of the alveolar margin or there appears to be undue resistance, the situation should be re-assessed with radiographs. The retained portion may vary in size from a whole root to a tiny apex. It may have broken either before or after there was movement of the tooth. The first decision to be made is whether the root should be left or extracted. There is little doubt that all pieces over 3 mm in length, or those which are non-vital or loose in the socket and might behave as foreign bodies, should be removed. This procedure may be contraindicated if the root lies near some important structure which could be damaged or if there are special medical considerations. Fractured roots of teeth extracted for orthodontic treatment should be removed. Where the orthodontist wishes to move teeth into the extraction site every effort must be made to conserve alveolar bone for this purpose. Whenever it is thought unnecessary or unwise to extract the roots they should be radiographed, the fact noted in the records and *the patient must always be told of their presence.*

Some roots can be seen by direct vision and the operator may decide he can apply elevators or forceps to them successfully through the socket, but often the very limited access makes this difficult and such manipulations can cause considerable trauma to bone and soft tissues. Where the retained fragments cannot be seen by direct vision it is bad surgical practice to attempt them 'blind' and an open or transalveolar approach is required.

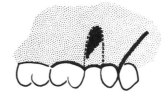

Fig. 8.10 Incision for flap for transalveolar approach.

The transalveolar approach

This is used to facilitate the extraction of retained roots or teeth which are considered difficult to extract or prove resistant to normal application of forceps or elevators. The surgeon must make a step-by-step plan for this operation, analysing carefully the size of flap, amount of bone removal and the point of application required to deliver the tooth or root satisfactorily.

A mucoperiosteal flap is raised to expose the alveolar bone enclosing the retained root. The incision should start at least the width of one tooth behind the root and maybe carried as far forward again. Where standing teeth are present it is made in the gingival crevice. From its anterior end the incision is then cut obliquely forwards and up or down into the buccal sulcus (Fig. 8.10). It is designed to avoid dividing the interdental papilla between standing teeth and should lie firmly supported on bone after the root has been removed. Another oblique incision posteriorly may be required to provide adequate access.

Bone is then removed to expose the root for a few millimetres to provide a new point of application for an elevator mesially, distally or buccally, and to obtain an unobstructed line of withdrawal. An elevator can be used to remove the root. For larger roots a Cryer's elevator can be satisfactorily applied buccally by drilling a hole into the root with a fissure bur at the level of the remaining alveolar bone. This is directed towards the apex at an angle of 45° to allow the elevator a greater range of upward movement (Fig. 8.11d). Sometimes, where there is hypercementosis or an apical hook, bone may have to be removed down to the apex to free it, care being taken not to expose the roots of neighbouring teeth.

Palatal roots of upper molars do present a problem. When approached buccally it is necessary to remove both the outer alveolar plate and their inter-radicular bone on the buccal aspect of the palatal socket. This gives good access and is a safe approach if the maxillary sinus does not dip down between the roots, but is very extravagant of alveolar bone. A palatal approach is advocated by some but it is more difficult to see into the wound and the bone is quite thick over the apical third of the root. An intra-alveolar approach is probably the best, the interseptal bone between palatal and buccal roots being slowly removed with burs till the root is exposed and an elevator can be used to draw it down.

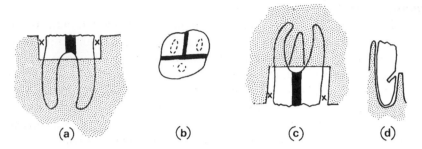

Fig. 8.11 (a) Division of roots of a lower tooth. (b) and (c) Division of upper molar roots. (d) Hole cut to apply Cryer's elevator to buccal aspect of a tooth. Note the angle of the cut to give maximum 'lift' to the root.

Where the whole of a difficult tooth or all the roots of an upper or lower molar tooth are retained, the buccal bone should be removed at least to the level of the bifurcation to allow forceps or elevators to be used. A Cryer's elevator may be applied buccally at the bifurcation to lift the roots. In many cases the radiographs will show them to have an unfavourable curvature which requires them to be divided and to be extracted separately (Fig. 8.11). This may be done with a fissure bur. Teeth must not be divided unless they have been exposed sufficiently to leave an adequate point of application on what remains of the roots after division.

A strong word of warning is necessary on two matters. First, the use of elevators on single retained roots which are in close relation to the maxillary sinus, or floor of the nose. *Upward pressure must not be used* even to gain a point of application, as this may cause the root to be displaced into one of these cavities. Bone should be gently removed to expose the root on one surface and downward movements only employed to extract it. In the mandible the inferior dental canal may present a similar hazard. Second, wherever flaps are being raised or bone removed near to the mental foramen the mental nerve must always be found, and preserved. In this respect bone-cutting should be severely limited in the vicinity of this structure.

Removal of roots after the socket has healed

The dental surgeon may be required to extract buried roots as a preparation for dentures, or because they are believed to be a source of pain or sepsis.

Localising roots

Once more, diagnosis and assessment is all-important if minimal damage is to be inflicted on the alveolar bone. The first step is to localise the root accurately with two radiographs at right angles to each other; both intraoral apical and occlusal views are required.

Removal of roots

The principles for removal of old retained roots are the same as for newly fractured teeth. In edentulous jaws the flap may be difficult to reflect and the horizontal incision is best made *just buccal* to the alveolar crest where the mucous
membrane is less tightly bound down. Where root apices are deeply placed it is
possible to make a curved incision in the alveolus away from the crest of the
ridge and remove the fragments through this. Bone is removed sparingly and
large roots may be divided to bring the occlusal portion apically as every
attempt must be made to spare the denture-bearing ridge.

Arrest of haemorrhage

After extracting teeth haemorrhage is arrested by asking the patient to bite
gently but firmly on the rolled up gauze swab placed over the socket. The buccal
and lingual gingival margins of the sockets must not be displaced outward by
the swab as this may lead to more bleeding. Should this not stop after ten
minutes, digital pressure is applied to the margins of the socket to localise the
bleeding point and to confirm that it can be stopped by pressing the gum against
the bone. Where this is effective simple interrupted or horizontal mattress
sutures are placed across the socket to draw the buccal and lingual alveolar
mucoperiosteum together. Though sutures closing an incision should not be tied
tightly, an exception is post-extraction haemorrhage where the soft tissues must
be firmly drawn against the bone. Tight suturing of this kind is contraindicated
where a defective clotting mechanism (as in haemophilia) may result in large
haemotomas forming in the tissue spaces if the blood is prevented from escap-
ing into the mouth.

Agents assisting haemostasis

Vasoconstrictors such as adrenalin 1:1000 in distilled water have been applied
topically to bleeding wounds. Their use is contraindicated for two reasons. First,
once the local effect has worn off it is not unusual to have a reactionary haemorrhage. Second, excess use may result in absorption of appreciable quantities
of the adrenalin to give systemic pressure symptoms.

Certain agents assist the physiological clotting mechanism. The most important is thrombin which acts on fibrinogen to form fibrin. Either human or bovine
varieties are available and may be applied topically either as a powder or as
an aqueous solution on gauze. Tranexamic acid mouthwash (10%) is advocated
and helps to prevent fibrinolysis. It has been used successfully to maintain
haemostasis in patients taking warfarin.

Mechanical agents, which include fibrin foam, gelatin foam, oxidised cellulose
and oxidised regenerated cellulose, are substances which form a water wettable

meshwork and assist clot formation. In general surgery they appear to be readily absorbed from wounds. In oral surgery the use of oxidised cellulose can give effective clot support and is resorbed with only few complications.

Post-extraction instructions

The incidence of post-extraction haemorrhage may be reduced by clear post-extraction instructions (Table 2.1). The patient must be warned not to use a mouthwash for the first 24 hours and thereafter normal oral hygiene may be resumed. Very hot or cold foods, alcohol or exercise are best avoided over the same period. Should bleeding occur he must sit up in bed or on a chair and bite on a rolled-up handkerchief. Where after half an hour these measures fail professional advice is required and he must be given the telephone number and address at which he can contact the dental surgeon. Where extractions were performed under a local anaesthetic the danger of biting or burning the anaesthetised lips or mouth should be stressed, particularly to children.

Further reading

Howe, G.L. (1980) *The Extraction of Teeth*, 2nd edn. Wrights & Sons, Bristol.

Chapter 9
Extraction of Unerupted or Partly Erupted Teeth

- Diagnosis
- Treatment
- Extraction of the impacted lower third molar
- Extraction of the upper third molar
- Extraction of the unerupted maxillary canine
- Extraction of maxillary supernumary teeth
- Other unerupted teeth

Teeth fail to erupt for many reasons. Evolutionary and hereditary factors which result in a disproportion in size between teeth and jaws are important. Local causes include retention or premature loss of a deciduous predecessor, the presence of supernumerary teeth, abnormal position of or injury to the tooth germ. Tumours and cysts may also prevent teeth from erupting. Certain conditions such as cleft palate, cleidocranial dysostosis, hypopituitarism, cretinism, rickets and facial hemiatrophy predispose to delay or failure of eruption.

The teeth most commonly concerned are the mandibular and maxillary third molars, and the maxillary canine. Others not infrequently seen are the mandibular second premolar and canine, the maxillary central incisors, and supernumerary teeth in both jaws. Many unerupted teeth are impacted – that is, prevented from erupting completely by other teeth or bone. Thus the lower third molar tooth commonly impacts against the second permanent molar.

Reasons for treatment

The majority of unerupted teeth are extracted because they give rise to symptoms of pain or become foci of infection. Other indications for removal are involvement in pathology such as cysts or tumours, evidence of causing resorption of roots of adjacent teeth, and interference in lines of osteotomies or fractures. Infection is less commonly seen in patients over 30 years old. The removal of asymptomatic unerupted teeth is not justified due to the possible sequelae of the surgery. This is particularly important when considering mandibular premolars and molars where the inferior dental and lingual nerves are at risk. Symptomless unerupted or partly erupted teeth should be monitored at intervals to detect the development of complications as outlined above.

Diagnosis

The diagnosis of unerupted teeth is based on the history, clinical examination and radiographs.

History

In the absence of infection the patient often has no complaint other than that a tooth is missing. The crown may cause a symptomless swelling under the mucosa. Where pain is thought to be a symptom from a completely buried tooth every effort must be made to eliminate other possible causes particularly pulpitis from another tooth.

Where infection is present more acute symptoms supervene. Inflammation about the crown of an unerupted or partly unerupted tooth is known as pericoronitis and is particularly serious when it arises from a lower third molar owing to the tendency of the infection to spread into the neck (Chapter 12).

Examination

The dentition is accurately charted for missing permanent teeth, retained deciduous teeth, caries and periodontal disease. Caries in a neighbouring tooth can often be the actual cause of the patient's symptoms of pain or infection, or may influence the plan of treatment where extraction of the carious tooth may allow the unerupted one to come into the space. Vitality tests of all doubtful teeth are essential. The unerupted tooth may displace, loosen, or resorb the roots of adjacent teeth against which it impacts. A cyst may form in association with the crown of the buried tooth. The mouth is examined for signs of infection such as swelling, discharge, trismus and enlarged tender lymph nodes.

Radiography

The object is to show the whole of the unerupted tooth, the size of its crown and the shape of its roots together with the direction in which they curve. The presence of hypercementosis or widening of the root particularly in the apical third is noted. In multirooted teeth the number of roots and whether they are fused or divergent is important. The position of the tooth in the jaws and its relationship to other teeth including the degree of impaction are an indication of the difficulty of the operation. Secondary conditions such as caries, an increase in the size of the follicle or resorption of adjacent tooth roots or of bone, will all affect the treatment plan (Fig. 9.1).

Radiographs in two planes at right angles to one another are required to show clearly the position of the tooth and the degree of impaction

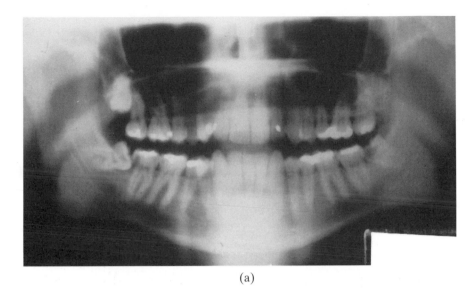

(a)

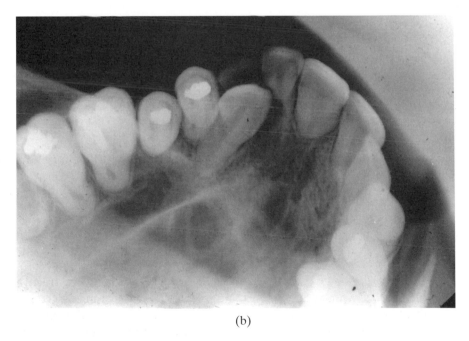

(b)

Fig. 9.1 (a) Impacted third molars; caries in lower left third molar and lower right second molar; (b) Impacted canine causing resorption of lateral incisor; (c) Retained deciduous canine and resorbed lateral incisor.

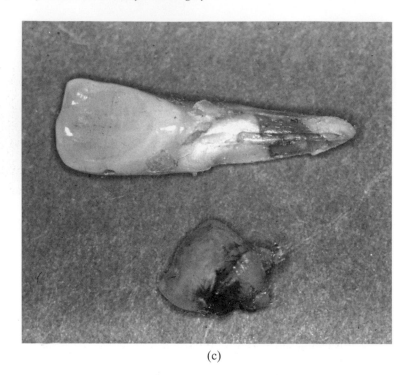

(c)

Fig. 9.1   (Continued).

(Fig. 9.2). The orthopantomograph is useful as a whole mouth scan where multiple unerupted teeth may be present.

Mandibular teeth

In the mandible localisation of unerupted teeth must show the whole tooth, its relationship to the inferior dental neurovascular bundle, its buccolingual position, and the relationship to adjacent teeth and the lower border of the mandible. The orthopantomograph is useful to show the position of the inferior dental neurovascular bundle and the depth of the mandible. For lower third molars this may be supplemented by an intraoral periapical film which shows more accurately the morphology of the tooth and its relationship to the second molar. To be of clinical value the radiograph must be correctly taken. The periapical film is placed with the upper border level and parallel with the occlusal plane of the second molar. The central ray is directed so that the buccal and lingual cusps of the second molar are superimposed one upon the other. The contact point between the first and second molars should be clearly shown without overlapping if the central ray has been correctly directed. This ensures that the film shows the true situation at the contact point between the third and second molar teeth, particularly how heavily the former is impacted. The distal bone over the crown of the unerupted tooth should be included. An occlusal film will show the bucco-

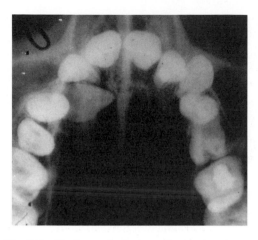
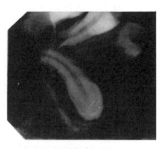

Fig. 9.2 Radiographs in two planes showing position of unerupted upper right canine. Occlusal view shows crown is palatally placed.

lingual positions of buried teeth. It is indicated for those teeth which lie across the arch, such as premolars. It is a difficult radiograph to take for third molars.

Deeply placed teeth or those lying in the ascending ramus cannot be seen on intraoral films and if not clearly seen on the orthopantomograph lateral oblique extraoral views may be indicated. These may also be used where there is an extensive secondary condition such as dentigerous cyst or where the mandible is very thin as in elderly edentulous patients.

Where the crown of the third molar tooth has not obviously erupted clear of bone it may be difficult to see on the radiographs exactly how the crown and distal bone are related. If the line of the anterior border of the ascending ramus distal to the third molar is projected to join the margin of the alveolar bone round the second molar, it will give a fair indication of the depth of overlying bone (Fig. 9.3).

Maxillary teeth

Intraoral periapical and occlusal films are both used in the diagnosis of unerupted maxillary teeth. The maxillary canine may need several periapical films to cover the whole of its length and its relationship to the adjacent teeth. Its position relative to the dental arch is important as it may be placed palatally, buccally, or more rarely across the arch. The only radiograph which will establish the true position of the canine in this respects is the vertex occlusal view taken with the central ray passing through the long axis of the incisor teeth (Fig. 9.2). This film will also show how close the unerupted canine lies to these teeth and may reveal curvatures of its root not obvious on the periapical view.

Alternatively the parallax method of Clark is used. In this, two periapical radiographs are taken with the films in the same position but with the X-ray

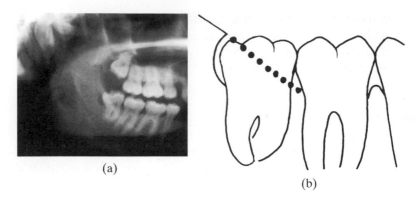

(a)

(b)

Fig. 9.3 Projection of bone over lower third molar. The dotted line in (b) is a projection of the anterior border of the ascending ramus extended to join the margin of the alveolar bone distal to the second molar, indicating that the distal cusp of the third molar is just covered by bone.

tube moved horizontally 3 cm in a known direction between exposures (that is from 1.5 cm behind the normal centring point to 1.5 cm in front of it). Where two teeth lie in different planes the one which appears to move in the same direction as the X-ray tube lies furthest from it, that is palatally. In analysing these radiographs the relationship of the crown and the root of the buried tooth to the roots of the standing teeth must be considered separately.

The true position of the unerupted tooth in the vertical dimension is not accurately shown on a periapical film because of the angle at which the ray is directed onto the maxilla. The orthopantomograph may provide a more satisfactory answer and will show unerupted teeth high in the maxilla related to the maxillary sinus. In teeth lying buccal to the arch a tangential view of the maxilla may be of assistance. Other unerupted maxillary teeth, supernumerary teeth and mesiodens are examined radiographically in much the same way.

Summary of findings

From his investigations the dental surgeon should know the following facts about the patient and the unerupted tooth. The patient's age, general development and the state of the dentition; the size and form of the crown of the unerupted tooth; whether it is resorbed or, in partly erupted teeth, carious; the form of the roots, fused or divergent, straight or curved mesially or distally. The position of the tooth in the bone, whether it is lying vertically, horizontally or inverted, how deeply it is buried in bone and its buccolingual or palatal relation to the arch. The relationship of the tooth to other teeth and to vital structures such as nerves, the nose and the maxillary sinus. The size of the follicle which may have atrophied, making extraction more difficult, undergone cystic change or have become infected. The texture of the bone, signs of osteosclerosis or in edentulous patients the degree of resorption of the mandible. The state of the adjoining teeth, whether caries, periodontal disease, apical areas or root resorption are present. With these facts established treatment may now be considered.

Treatment

Treatment may be conservative, to bring the tooth into useful occlusion in the arch, or removal, or the tooth may be left *in situ* but kept under review.

Conservative treatment

Conservative treatment should be considered for patients where the tooth might be brought into occlusion. The advice of a specialist orthodontist is necessary as orthodontic treatment may be required prior to surgery to create space in the arch for the unerupted tooth. A conservative approach is particularly important where a neighbouring standing tooth is carious or heavily filled. In some cases eruption may not take place without exposure of the tooth and the use of traction.

Exposure of teeth

To expose teeth a mucoperiosteal flap is made and bone is removed with burs to free the crown down to its greatest circumference. For incisors and canines the cingulum must be exposed. Every precaution should be taken to avoid dislodging the tooth accidentally. Where the orthodontist wants a bracket, or other device to apply traction, this is placed at operation. For palatally placed teeth the soft tissues are then excised round the crown and the dead space packed with Coepack or Whitehead's varnish on gauze. These are removed after ten days when the patient should be referred back to the orthodontist. Care must be taken with exposure of buccally placed teeth for there is evidence that excision of the soft tissues back to non-keratinised mucosa results in an unsatisfactory epithelial cuff around the erupted tooth. Many orthodontists prefer to apply a bracket to such teeth with a wire brought out through the wound for traction. The mucoperiosteal flap is then sutured back into position.

Surgical repositioning and transplantion

In both these techniques the tooth, after exposure, is moved bodily to bring it into the dental arch. In surgical repositioning the tooth is rotated through an angle which must be less than 90° to prevent damage to the apical vessels. In transplantation the tooth is carefully extracted and placed in a surgically prepared socket. It is immobilised with a splint for about 4 weeks, when it is usually firm. The teeth most frequently transplanted are unerupted maxillary canines replanted into their correct position and third molars used to replace carious first molars. Good results are obtained with young patients, but resorption of roots is a complication after 2–5 years which occasionally leads to loss of the tooth. Early endodontic treatment may help to prevent this.

Extraction of unerupted teeth

If the decision has been made to remove an unerupted tooth this is best accomplished before it is complicated by sclerosis of bone, atrophy of the follicle which reduces the free space round the crown, or by the presence of infection. The roots when fully formed frequently develop hooked or bulbous apices and in adults the impaction of the crown against adjoining teeth is often severe.

Ideally the tooth is removed when the roots are two-thirds complete; before this the crown may be difficult to elevate as it tends to turn in its socket like the ball in a ball-and-socket joint. Removal of a symptomless tooth is best postponed if it is acting as a buttress for the root of an adjacent tooth which may be simultaneously bereft of support and denuded of bone.

It is also contraindicated where vital structures such as the inferior dental nerve may be damaged in the course of the operation. In acute pericoronitis, surgery may have to be delayed due to difficulties in opening the mouth.

Planning the operation

This is best done by considering first the position of the tooth in the jaw, second its natural line of withdrawal, third the obstacles to its extraction and how these may best be overcome, forth the points of application for elevators, and finally access by removing bone and raising the flap sufficient to allow the necessary procedures to be performed.

Thus the plan is made in the reverse order to that in which the operation will be performed, as obviously the size and form of the flap depends on bone removal and this in turn is related to the position of the tooth and any manoeuvres required to disimpact it.

Natural line of withdrawal

This may be shown on radiographs by projecting the line along which the tooth would move if it followed the course dictated by the curvature of its roots. Teeth are most easily extracted by moving them out of their sockets or out of bone along this pathway. Where the tooth would come through the alveolus into the mouth unimpeded, except by alveolar bone, it is said to be favourably placed, but where it would go deeper into bone or impact against another tooth it is classified as unfavourable.

Extraction by moving the teeth along their line of withdrawal is done with elevators, using a gentle touch and always watching the effect of the forces applied to the tooth or roots. Heavy levering either to disimpact the tooth or lift it from its socket may have serious consequences such as fracture of the bone, or displacement of the tooth into the soft tissues or the maxillary sinus. Where the roots of mandibular teeth are near the inferior dental canal this nerve may be damaged. Resistance to elevation should be foreseen and plans made to overcome it.

Obstacles to elevation of a tooth

These may occur along its natural line of withdrawal and may be 'intrinsic', that is due to the shape of the tooth, such as hooked or bulbous apices, roots curving in opposite directions or a constriction at the neck of the tooth, all of which may anchor the tooth in bone. As many of these difficulties are found in the apical third of the root considerable bone removal may be necessary to free the tooth.

The obstacles may also be 'extrinsic', that is due to bone, adjacent teeth or vital structures such as the inferior dental nerve or the maxillary antrum. The depth of the tooth in bone is a major factor in assessing difficulty, presenting problems of access, increasing the time of operation, and requiring foresight and experience to avoid excessive bone destruction.

Where the unerupted tooth is impacted against other teeth which are not for extraction its disimpaction is usually a simple problem in geometry. The tooth may be extracted whole by removing sufficient bone to allow it to be rotated, and this is often possible (Fig. 9.4a). Where the impaction is severe (Fig. 9.4e) or the root curvature adverse (Fig. 9.4b) it must be divided and extracted in pieces. This is a less traumatic and safer method than forceful levering to disimpact the tooth and preserves bone which may later form part of the edentulous denture-bearing ridge. Division may be horizontal (crown from roots, Fig. 9.4e) or vertical (down the long axis of the tooth, Fig. 9.4d). Both are preferably done with a large bur, to leave an appreciable space between the divided parts. A hole is made through the centre of the root below the amelocemental junction with a no. 7 fissure bur. To divide the crown from the roots the cut is extended mesially and distally through the whole thickness of the tooth. The angle of cut is important and should be made to favour the line of withdrawal of the crown (Figs 9.4 and 9.5). Wherever the tooth is related to any important structure a thick layer of dentine is left intact and the last portion cracked through by rotating an elevator in the cut. Division with an osteotome is less satisfactory as it produces a hair-line crack, often at the wrong angle, which makes disimpaction of the crown very difficult. When it is used, the tooth must be firmly supported in bone and not loose; the osteotome is applied to the cementum and given a sharp blow with the mallet.

Division vertically is reserved for molar teeth, particularly those with divergent roots, and is very effective in certain impactions (Fig. 9.4d). It is obviously ineffective where the roots are fused or the cut misses their bifurcation. Removal of part of the crown may leave a convenient point of application for an elevator; which is crucial for success in distoangular impaction. (Fig. 9.4c).

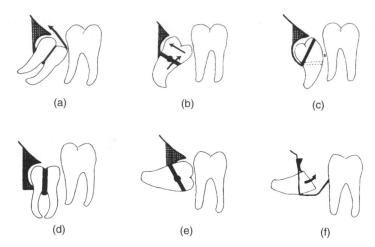

Fig. 9.4 The disto-buccal bone to be removed is shown by cross-hatching. (a) Mesioangular impaction with favourable roots. The tooth may rotate about the distal apex but may require division as shown and the roots elevated separately. (b) Mesioangular impaction with unfavourable roots requiring division. (c) Distoangular impaction with oblique division to maintain mesial point of application. (d) Vertical impaction with separate roots may require vertical division. (e) Horizontal impaction: note angle of division of crown to allow removal of divided fragment. (f) The roots can then be elevated forwards.

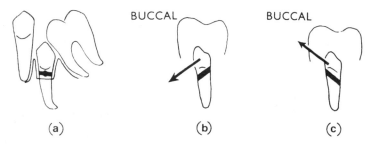

Fig. 9.5 Impacted second premolar: (a) bone removal, and division of tooth: (b) correct buccolingual angulation of the dividing cut; (c) incorrect angulation as crown cannot disimpact from the first molar.

Point of application for elevators

Dental elevators when properly used are very sensitive instruments through which even the slightest resistance to movement of a tooth or root can be felt. For this reason they are the most satisfactory instrument for extracting buried teeth. It must be decided at the planning stage at which points it will be necessary to apply an elevator to lift the tooth, or after it has been divided the crown and then the roots, out of the socket. Bone may have to be removed with the sole object of obtaining satisfactory access or a fulcrum for the elevator. Tooth division must be planned so that after removal of the crown enough root is exposed to enable elevators to be applied easily. No tooth should be divided until an adequate point of application on the fraction that is to be left in bone has been prepared and tested, otherwise the operator's difficulties may be greatly increased by this injudicious action.

Access

Only after all the above factors have been considered can the full extent of bone removal be calculated. Inadequate access is the commonest cause of difficulty in the extraction of unerupted teeth. The flap must be sufficiently large to allow direct vision into the whole field. Bone removal should permit the greatest circumference of the crown to pass freely out of the bone along the planned line of withdrawal and provide access for dividing the tooth if necessary. Where the greatest diameter of the roots is not at the neck of the tooth, the bulbous section must be made free of bone. The cutting of bone should not be punctuated by hopeful attempts to extract the tooth, but is completed as one stage of the operation before elevation is tried. Indeed the preparation of satisfactory access for elevators and of a fulcrum on firm bone offering them adequate support is an important part of planned bone removal.

The size and shape of the flap in its turn depends on the extent of the operation as it must provide access without subjecting the soft tissues to tension or trauma. The flap must extend beyond the area of bone removal so that the line of closure rests on bone (Fig. 9.6).

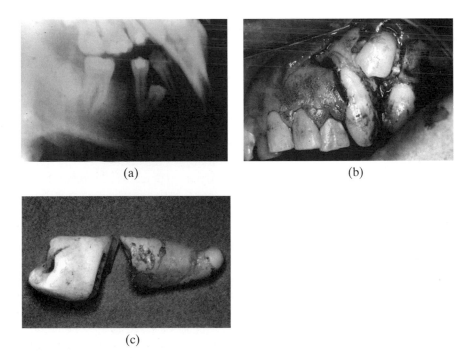

(a)

(b)

(c)

Fig. 9.6 Unerupted lower first premolar: (a) radiographic appearance; (b) buccal mucosa reflected to reveal position; (c) division required to remove tooth.

Teeth in edentulous jaws

These often present in older patients when the bone is sclerotic and the peri-odontal space very narrow. The principles of removal are similar to those described, but it may be necessary to cut a point of application for an elevator and very gentle forces should be applied as the bone is brittle. Special care is taken to preserve the alveolar ridge by making an accurate assessment and removing minimal bone. Where gross resorption of the mandible has taken place, and there is danger of fracturing the jaw, the patient should be warned and a suitable plating kit should be available (Chapter 14).

Closure

Debridement is completed in the normal way and the flap reapposed. Sutures, which may be resorbable, should be kept to a minimum. If the design of flap allows primary closure of the wound then this should be achieved as long as the flap is not under tension.

Extraction of the impacted lower third molar

Assessment

Position of the tooth and its line of withdrawal

The position of the unerupted lower third molar may be vertical (Fig. 9.4d), hori-zontal (Fig. 9.4e), mesioangular (Fig. 9.4a) or distoangular (Fig. 9.4c). The crown usually lies nearer the lingual than the buccal plate. Occasionally it is inverted or lies across the mandible, with the crown facing either bucally or lingually. Very rarely it is found in the ascending ramus or at the lower border of the mandible. Where the tooth lies below the inferior dental canal an extraoral lower border approach is indicated.

The natural line of the tooth can only be determined by a study of radi-ographs showing the form of the roots which may be fused, divergent, straight or curved to favour or prevent extraction of the tooth.

The difficulty of the extraction is increased if access is difficult. This may occur if the mouth is small, where the space between the anterior border of the mandible and the distal aspect of the second molar is narrow or when the tooth is deeply buried in bone.

Obstacles to extraction

Bone

All or part of the crown may be covered by bone (Fig. 9.3). How deeply the tooth is buried is calculated by measuring the vertical distance from the cervi-cal margin of the second molar to the mesial cervical margin of the tooth except in distoangular impactions where the distal cervical margin is used. Where this distance is over 4mm the tooth should be regarded as deeply buried. Vertically placed buried teeth may only need bone to be removed from over the whole of the occlusal and buccal surfaces of the crown for them to be elevated up and out with a Cryer's elevator applied to the buccal aspect of the root.

They must, however, be distinguished from the tooth that is distally impacted against the bone of the ascending ramus. These are the most difficult of all impacted third molars to extract. They should always be approached with great caution, especially where they are deeply placed, lie far back in the ascending ramus, or the roots have a distal curvature (Fig. 9.4c).

After removal of buccal and occlusal bone to clear the crown the tooth should be divided, the crown removed, and using a point of application on the buccal aspect of the roots they are elevated into the space created.

Where the roots are curved distally this may still prove difficult until further bone has been cut to free them distally, or the roots are sectioned again. If the roots are separate vertical division is often useful.

The inferior dental neurovascular bundle

This may be damaged by direct trauma from burs or elevators, or indirectly when the tooth is elevated or rotated as the root can crush or tear the neurovascular bundle.

The relationship of roots, particularly of the lower third molar, to the inferior dental canal may be deduced from radiographs. It may clearly lie below the roots or appear to cross them. In the latter relationship it is probably grooving the roots if the radiolucent band of the canal is seen to cross them above their apices. Where the root is deeply notched the white lines, representing the cortical plates lining the canal, converge, are diverted or are interrupted (Fig. 9.7). This is a warning that heavy or repeated elevation may compress the nerve against bone to cause hypoaesthesia or paraesthesia. Such damage can be avoided by planning the operation so that sufficient bone is removed and, where

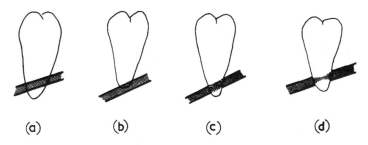

Fig. 9.7 Relationship of the third molar roots to the inferior dental canal as seen on radiographs: (a) root lightly notched; (b) apical notch; (c) deeply notched; (d) the canal perforates the root.

indicated, the tooth divided to allow the roots to be lifted out with a single gentle movement.

Perforation of a root by the canal contents is suggested where the radiolucent band crosses the root and shows the loss of both white lines with maximum constriction of the radiolucent band at the middle of the root (Fig. 9.7d). The tooth must then be divided, and removed from around the nerve or, where this is not possible, the nerve is cut with a sharp scalpel and the ends replaced in the canal, following which, sensation often returns after a few months.

Impaction against a tooth

The third molar may impact against the second molar either in the mesioanglar (Fig. 9.4a) or in the horizontal position (Fig. 9.4e). The impaction may be overcome in one of three ways.

Extraction of the second molar can be justified by gross caries or periodontal disease. It is often advised where the third molar is heavily impacted against the distal root of the second molar without any apparent intervening alveolar bone. This should not be necessary if the surgeon avoids damaging the second molar roots and the soft tissue round the neck of that tooth. Usually the second molar is sound and the operation must be planned to protect it from damage during the extraction of the buried tooth.

Rotation of the impacted tooth, particularly if it is in a favourable mesioangular position, may allow it to be turned bodily away from the second molar. This can be planned on radiographs. The apex of the distal root of the third molar is taken as the centre of a circle through which the tooth might be rotated. A radius is drawn to the mesiobuccal cusp and if the arc of this circle passes clear of the second molar, then the third molar should disimpact without difficulty, providing sufficient bone can be removed distally to allow it to turn (Fig. 9.4a). This technique is often satisfactory for mesioangular impactions, but would require extensive bone removal for horizontal impactions. When assessing the tooth for rotation the relationship of the apex of the distal root to the inferior dental canal should be examined as rotation may force this apex downwards and if the canal is immediately below, the neurovascular bundle may be crushed with resulting anaesthesia or paraesthesia.

Division of the impacted tooth is indicated where the impaction is heavy, the curvature of the roots is unfavourable or where a large amount of bone would otherwise have to be removed. In horizontal impactions bone is removed from the buccal and upper surface of the crown and coronal third of the root. The tooth is then divided through the neck, using an oblique cut (Fig. 9.4e) so that the crown may be easily disimpacted by sliding it up and back along the distally inclined plane on the root. The roots are then brought forward using a Cryer's elevator on their superior surface. Where the roots have a mesial unfavourable curvature or are divergent, difficulty may be experienced and further division of the roots may be necessary.

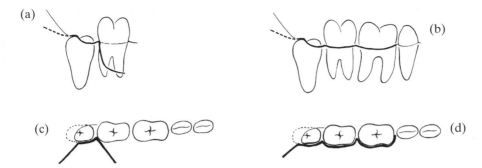

Fig. 9.8 Flaps for removal of unerupted third molar: (a) and (c) standard flap with distal relieving incision following external oblique ridge; (b) and (d) envelope flap with same distal extension as standard; further flexibility can be gained by lengthening the ginvial margin incision.

Operative technique

The flap

The incision for partly erupted third molars is commenced in the distal part of the gingival crevice and carried buccally round the crown of the tooth to just behind the crown of the second molar (where the tooth is buried the incision starts on the alveolar crest, distal to the second molar). It is then carried down and slightly anteriorly to the reflection where it is turned to run forward parallel to, but just above the reflection, stopping just short of the distal root of the first molar, to avoid a small artery at this point. Using a Mitchell's trimmer the edge of the flap is freed starting in the buccal sulcus and working distally. It may then be reflected with the Howarth's periosteal elevator to expose the external oblique line of the mandible. The incision is then continued along this line and up the ascending ramus using either scissors or a scalpel on the anterior edge of the ramus where the flap will fall away from the bone easily and small vessels are avoided (Fig. 9.8).

The envelope flap

The incision is carried forward in the gingival crevice of the second and first molar teeth and relieved distal to the third molar towards the external oblique ridge. Initially the flap is raised along the gingival margin with a suitable fine instrument such as a flat plastic or a curved Warwick James elevator to avoid damage to the margin (Fig. 9.8b).

Both of the above flaps should give adequate access to remove bone from the buccal aspect only. Lingual retraction is not advocated as it may cause damage to the lingual nerve. If a lingual flap is necessary this should be raised with extreme care distal to the third molar ensuring the instrument is below the periosteum to avoid damage to the lingual nerve.

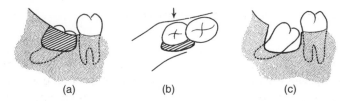

Fig. 9.9   Disto-buccal bone removal for third molar removal: (a) bone should be removed vertically around the crown (shaded area); (b) from above it can be seen that bone should not be removed toward the disto-lingual aspect; (c) at the end of bone removal the bifurcation area should be exposed. This will facilitate division of the tooth as indicated in Fig. 9.4.

Bone removal

With the improvement in high speed drills incorporating water delivery systems bone removal is now almost universally achieved using burs. Bone can quickly be removed by grinding using a tungsten carbide rosehead bur.

Sufficient bone should be removed to allow the tooth to be elevated without the use of undue force. In general the whole of the buccal aspect of the crown as far as the bifurcation should be exposed (Fig. 9.9). This facilitates tooth division which, as discussed previously, may be essential to enable the tooth to be elevated more easily. Care should be taken not to destroy the application points for elevators by injudicious division. This can usually be achieved by removing bone only from the buccal aspect of the tooth.

Horizontally impacted teeth may then be divided whereas mesioangular teeth are disimpacted using a no. 1 Coupland's elevator or a straight Warwick James elevator placed mesially at the neck of the tooth, and rotated to move it distally and buccally; it is then lifted out of its socket with a Cryer's elevator used mesially or buccally in the bifurcation of the roots.

Debridement

The wound must be cleansed of debris and the follicle of the tooth removed by grasping it firmly in tissue forceps and drawing it gently off the bone. Where it is attached to the flap, this may be gently dissected off with a Mitchell's trimmer, but great care should be taken on the lingual side as the lingual nerve may be inadvertently damaged.

Closure

One suture in the distal part of the incision, over the external oblique ridge, is usually sufficient to hold the flap in position. Primary closure of the wound edges can protect the socket and improve the chances of uneventful healing but the flap should not be placed under tension to achieve this as it will tend to break down.

Extraction of the upper third molar tooth

Assessment

Access is made difficult by the position of the upper third molar behind the second molar, the presence of the malar buttress, and the way in which the coronoid process comes forward when the mouth is open. Fortunately, the majority are buccally placed and covered by only a thin layer of bone.

Their roots vary widely in form but they are often small and fine and fracture easily. The roots, and sometimes the whole tooth, are commonly in close relation to the maxillary sinus into which they can be displaced. Deeply placed distoangular teeth can easily be pushed into the soft tissue behind the maxillary tuberosity. Upper third molars seldom give trouble whilst buried and in view of this there is a strong argument for leaving those that are symptomless to erupt or until the second molar is to be extracted. Erupted upper third molars which are functionless may be extracted at the same time as the lower third molar.

The flap

The incision is made from the distal aspect of the maxillary tuberosity forward to the middle of the distal aspect of the second molar crown. This part of the incision should be kept over towards the palate to expose the third molar without raising a second palatal flap which is often difficult to retract and may cause retching in some patients. The incision is then carried obliquely forward into the buccal sulcus in a similar fashion to the design of the lower third molar. The flap is reflected and held back with the periosteal elevator (Fig. 9.10).

Bone removal

The bone over this tooth is usually quite thin and can be removed with burs or with a sharp chisel used with gentle pressure by hand to avoid accidentally pushing the tooth into the maxillary sinus. When the occlusal, buccal and distal aspect of the crown have been exposed an elevator (Cryer's or Warwick James) may be applied to the buccal surface of this tooth to bring it *downwards*. Mesioangular impactions may be disimpacted from behind the upper second molar with an elevator. In either case a Howarth's raspatory must be placed distally to prevent the tooth being luxated backward into the soft tissues (Fig. 9.10).

Extraction of the unerupted maxillary canine

Assessment

The unerupted maxillary canine may lie palatally, bucally or across the dental arch between the roots of the standing teeth. In this last case the root apex or the crown may be palpated in the buccal sulcus. Some are deeply placed high

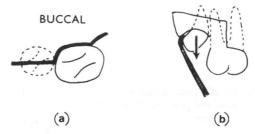

Fig. 9.10   (a) Design of buccal flap for upper third molar. Note that the distal extension of the incision over the tuberosity is carried well over towards the palatal side. (b) Extraction of upper third molar with a Howarth's raspatory placed behind the tooth to prevent it displacing backwards into the soft tissue spaces.

up in the maxilla or in the floor of the nose. The tooth may be in vertical, mesioangular, distoangular, or horizontal impaction; rarely it is inverted. Many unerupted canines have curved roots often sharply hooked in the apical third.

Radiographs in two planes must be carefully examined to localise the tooth, to determine its relationship to the dental arch and to detect the site and direction of any curvature of the roots (Fig. 9.2). The relationship of the canine to the standing teeth is most important, particularly for palatally placed canines which may in fact have caused so much resorption of alveolar bone that they are supporting the teeth against which they are impacted. Wherever the impaction is close, or the standing teeth have been moved or show signs of resorption by the canine, vitality tests should be carried out, and splints prepared beforehand to support the standing teeth during and after operation.

In those canines lying in the arch between the roots of the standing teeth, tangential views of the maxilla are important in determining the position of the incisal tip, whether it is lying palatal or buccal to the arch. Where it has passed buccally between the roots of the teeth it is necessary to expose the crown buccally even though the tooth may have to be approached palatally as well.

It is a common fault for inexperienced surgeons to omit to make a stage-by-stage operation plan for unerupted canines, possibly because the approach to these teeth is less standardised than for the lower third molar. It is essential before starting, to be quite clear about the proposed line of withdrawal, the bone to be removed and the points of application to be prepared.

Buccally placed canines

These are extracted through a buccal incision, which is made in a long curve about 3 cm in length and at least half a centimetre above the gingival margin of the standing teeth. The thin layer of bone over the tooth is removed and it is gently eased outwards with a Cryer's elevator and, when it is disimpacted, extracted with forceps.

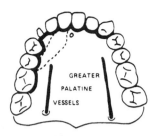

Fig. 9.11 Design of a palatal flap for extraction of a buried canine. Note the position of the incisive foramen and the palatine vessels.

Palatally placed canines

The flap

As the approach is through a palatal flap the field of operation is best seen if the surgeon works from the opposite side, that is the patient's left, for a tooth on the right. The incision is made in the gingival crevice round the necks of the standing teeth. For a tooth on the right side it extends from the upper left canine to the upper right first molar. The flap is reflected carefully to lift the mucoperiosteum containing the palatine artery without damaging that vessel. The structures passing through the incisive foramen may have to be divided as they restrict access (Fig. 9.11).

Where two canines are to be extracted the flap is best made from first molar to first molar. The flap can be held back with a retractor, a hook or by passing a suture through it tied to the teeth on the opposite side.

Bone removal

This should be done very accurately with a medium-sized rosehead bur (5–9) keeping *to the palatal side* of the buried tooth. Bone is removed till the crown is found; it is then cleared of bone particularly over the incisive tip and the coronal third of the root. Every effort must be made to *leave the supporting bone over the roots of the standing teeth* and to avoid accidentally cutting into their roots. Special care is needed where the canine lies across the arch.

Extraction

Many vertical canines with straight roots will elevate downwards once the crown is cleared. Others, particularly those in a horizontal position impacted against other teeth, should be divided and the crown extracted first. Elevators are best applied to the palatal side of the tooth or up its long axis. Occasionally, elevation from the buccal side is unavoidable. In these circumstances the fingers of the watching hand are placed over the standing teeth to detect even the slightest movement in them, and, where a splint has been constructed this may be put over the teeth to support them and removed after the extraction.

Great difficulty may be found when the apical third of the root is curved or hooked, particularly if this curvature is unfavourable and turns the tooth into the dental arch, making it necessary to remove bone from over its whole length to free the apex. Many canines are closely related to the maxillary sinus into which they can be displaced by forceful or misdirected application of elevators. Should a root apex which is known to be near the antrum fracture it is wise to consider leaving it.

Those teeth which lie across the dental arch with the crown in the palate and the root apex in the buccal sulcus may require a flap made both palatally and buccally. Where the apex of the root is hooked, division may be necessary to extract the apex bucally, and to allow the crown to be removed palatally which can often be done by firm pressure exerted through the buccal approach.

Closure

The palatal flap when replaced will require only one or two sutures to hold it. The knots should be tied buccally.

Osteoplastic flaps

Canines in edentulous jaws are often lying along the arch so that their removal may destroy the bony ridge and damage the denture bearing area. The ridge can be preserved by the use of an osteoplastic flap. Two buccal, vertical incisions are made just beyond the estimated position of the root apex and the incisal tip of the tooth. These are joined by an incision along the crest of the ridge. The margin, 3 mm only, of the buccal flap is reflected to admit a chisel or fissure bur which is used to make cuts through the bone parallel to the vertical and horizontal incisions. The latter must be on the crest of the ridge and cut up to the tooth. A Howarth's periosteal elevator is placed in this cut and rotated outwards so that the buccal bone fractures and, still attached to mucoperiosteum, is raised buccally (Fig. 9.12). The canine can then be seen and removed with an elevator. The osteoplastic flap is carefully replaced and the mucosa sutured. The bony ridge is thus preserved and the patient can often continue to wear the denture within alteration.

Extraction of maxillary supernumerary teeth

Supernumerary teeth in the incisor region of the maxilla are of common occurrence. They are diagnosed and operated in much the same way as unerupted maxillary canines. Where the supernumerary is associated with an unerupted incisor it is best extracted as soon as possible to avoid causing delayed or

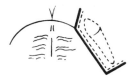 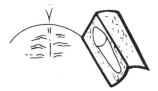

Fig. 9.12 Osteoplastic flap. Left: Continuous dark line indicates the incision through mucoperiosteum along the alveolar crest and extended obliquely upwards in the buccal mucoperiosteum anteriorly and posteriorly. Dashed line indicates limited extent of reflection of the flap to allow bone incision to be made. Right: Mucoperiosteum and bone flap reflected to expose canine tooth.

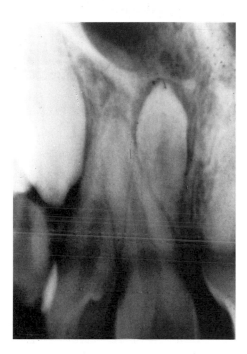

Fig. 9.13 Upper midline supernumerary (mesiodens). Note rotation of left central incisor.

arrested eruption. It is essential to expose clearly and identify the permanent teeth and the supernumerary *without doubt* before any form of elevation is started.

Other unerupted teeth

Other unerupted teeth in the maxilla and mandible will present their own problems to the surgeon which he must solve by applying the principles described above to each new situation.

Further reading

Dimitroulis, G. (1997) *A Synopsis of Minor Oral Surgery*. Wright, Oxford.

NHS Centre for reviews and dissemination. (1998) Prophylactic removal of impacted third molars: is it justified? *Effectiveness Matters*, **3**, issue 2.

Robinson, P.P. & Smith, K.G. (1996) Lingual nerve damage during lower third molar removal: a comparison of two surgical methods. *Brit. Dent. J.*, **180**(12), 456–61.

Rood, J.P. & Nooraldeen Shehab, B.A.A. (1990) The radiological prediction of damage to the inferior alveolar nerve during the extraction of mandibular third molar. *Brit. Dent. J.*, **109**, 335.

Chapter 10
Complications of Tooth Extraction

- Pre-extraction
- During extraction
- Post-extraction

Pre-extraction

Difficulty in achieving anaesthesia

Where breakdown in pain control is encountered during extraction careful diagnosis of the nerve distribution in which pain sensation remains is essential. The presence of collateral nerve supply must be anticipated and appropriate techniques such as periodontal ligament injection employed. Tooth extraction under local anaesthesia should be possible in almost all co-operative patients and the surgeon should strive to perfect techniques which ensure the procedure is painless.

Difficulty in co-operation

This may be encountered at any time during the procedure especially in those patients not amenable to reasoning, but careful pre-operative assessment should alert the surgeon to such problems. The surgeon should on no account force any patient to accept treatment and an alternative method of achieving the extraction should be sought with as little delay as possible. This might involve the use of sedation or general anaesthesia.

Difficulty of access

Trismus

Limitation of opening may be due to intrinsic causes (abnormalities in the temporomandibular joint) or extrinsic causes (facial scars and inflammatory swellings). In chronic cases it may be possible to improve the opening with exercisers, but forcing the jaws open when trismus is due to infection will break down the pyogenic membrane and cause spread. The acute phase is treated with antibiotics and drainage and the extractions delayed till the opening is sufficiently improved.

Reduced aperture of the mouth

This may be due to congenital malformation (microstomia) or to scarring, making it difficult or even impossible to apply forceps or elevators to the teeth. In extreme cases a surgical approach through the angle of the mouth may be necessary.

Crowded or misplaced teeth

These frequently make it difficult to apply forceps or elevators without the risk of loosening adjacent teeth. This may be made easier by dividing or grinding down, with discs or burs, the tooth to be extracted.

During extraction

Abnormal resistance

Where there is no obvious clinical cause for abnormal resistance such as the position of the tooth or the thickness of the alveolar bone, the operator should make steady and repeated efforts to loosen the tooth, avoiding too much force in one direction. After a reasonable attempt, if there is no movement, a radiograph is taken before proceeding further. This may show abnormalities of the roots in number or in form such as twisted, divergent, bulbous or hypercementosed roots. In age or chronic periodontal disease there may be sclerosis of the alveolar bone. Isolated teeth in occlusion are renownedly difficult to remove owing to narrowing of the periodontal membrane. Unerupted teeth impacting against the roots of the tooth to be extracted (lower third molar against second molar roots) can be a source of difficulty only discovered on a radiograph.

In all cases of abnormal resistance it is advisable to plan removal of the tooth through a transalveolar approach to reduce trauma and avoid fracturing the tooth.

Damage to other teeth

Extraction of the wrong tooth

This is a common source of litigation and is indefensible because it is avoidable if the proper precautions are taken. Extractions should never be started without checking *immediately* before operation, the patient's name, address and age, the teeth to be removed and any radiographs available. This applies equally to patients operated on under local or general anaesthesia. The patient, or in the case of children the parent, is asked to confirm he understands which teeth are to be extracted, and any doubts in his mind must be settled before the anaesthetic is given.

The notes should be placed so that the operator can see them throughout the operation and can make a final check just before the forceps are applied to the tooth. Should an error occur, the surgeon must proceed to extract the right tooth to complete the operation. He has then to decide whether to re-implant the wrongly extracted tooth immediately or to accept the situation.

Dislocation of adjacent teeth or of restorations in adjacent teeth

Careless application or movements of forceps and elevators may cause this mishap. Forceps can accidentally engage part of the next tooth and so loosen it, or when drawing a lower tooth from its socket without sufficient control they may bang against the upper teeth. Elevators, misused either as class I levers or by employing a neighbouring tooth, and not bone, as the fulcrum, can do similar damage. The watching fingers of the supporting hand can assist in preventing this by feeling that the forceps are in good position and detecting even slight movement in adjacent teeth. Where misplaced or mildly impacted teeth occur in the arch, a disc or bur should be used on the tooth to allow its extraction without transmitting pressure or force to its neighbours.

The permanent premolars may be luxated when extracting the deciduous molars due to the root formation of the deciduous teeth which may closely approximate the crown of the permanent tooth, or infection which may cause fibrosis or even ankylosis between them. More often it is due to the misapplication of instruments in the extraction of deciduous molars or injudicious attempts to remove their retained roots.

Fracture of teeth

Where normal extracting methods are used the teeth may fracture owing to advanced caries or large restorations which weaken the crown. In devitalised teeth, in periodontal disease and in the aged, the roots may become brittle, and it is unfortunate that the last two conditions are also characterised by sclerosis and loss of elasticity of the alveolar bone thereby causing undue resistance to add to the dentist's difficulties.

Another common cause is ill-fitting forceps which impinge on the crown or do not fit the root accurately. Forceps may be misapplied particularly on rotated, inclined or misplaced teeth. The use of excess force or short, jerky movements prevents the surgeon feeling which way the tooth wants to come and frequently results in fracture.

The management of retained roots has been discussed in Chapter 8. However, if certain principles are neglected the attempted removal of such roots may lead to more serious complications. It is essential that a radiograph should be taken and, except where the crown has fractured at or above the level of the alveolar margin, it is bad practice to use forceps up the socket as the limited access makes it difficult to open the beaks sufficiently to grasp the root. Only too often forceps are applied knowing that one or both blades are outside the alveolus which must be crushed to deliver the root. The transalveolar approach must always be used wherever the root is not clearly visible or supporting tissues will be damaged. It is safe, leaves the tissue in good condition, and, if regularly practised without delay, is economic in time.

Loss of tooth or roots

As the teeth and roots are extracted they should be carefully placed in a special container, care being taken not to carry them back into the mouth by accident. At the end of the operation, particularly under general anaesthesia, they should be counted and the number checked against the chart.

Where during extractions a tooth or root is lost, the surgeon should *immediately* stop operating and conduct a systematic search.

The mouth

All the recesses of the mouth, under the tongue and recent sockets are examined. In patients under general anaesthesia, the posterior aspect of the tongue and oropharynx are searched too. After this has been done the superficial layers of the throat pack may be drawn forward lest it be lying there. The pack should not be removed completely till the end of the operation.

Spittoon and suction apparatus

The spittoon should always have a trap, and the suction apparatus a bottle in the circuit to stop fragments of tooth disappearing down the drain. The sucker head, rubber tubing and other connections should be washed through as they often trap root apices.

Alimentary tract or lungs

Roots or teeth may be swallowed or inhaled. Whenever it is suspected that this may have happened radiographs of the chest or abdomen should be taken. Swallowed fragments seldom give cause for anxiety, though their passage through the gut should be monitored, but if inhaled into the lungs the patient must be referred, without delay, to a thoracic surgeon for removal by bronchoscopy.

Under the mucoperiosteum

Roots and occasionally teeth can be displaced under the periosteum particularly in the mandible where there has been gross recession of alveolar bone or flaps have been raised past the reflection of the mucous membrane. A finger should be placed at once below the root and kept there to prevent it going deeper. A flap may be raised to expose the root which can then be lifted out using a blunt hooked instrument. Attempts should not be made to grasp it with forceps as if they fail to grip the root they may drive it deeper into the space.

The tissue spaces

In the mandible, roots or teeth can be lost in the tissue spaces of the floor of the mouth either above or below the mylohyoid muscle. The lower third molar roots can be pushed down lingually through the bottom of the socket if this is deficient, as does occasionally occur; the root then lies below the mylohyoid. During the extraction of the unerupted lower third molar it can be elevated lingually into the tissue spaces. In all these cases the grave danger is that the tooth will pass into the deeper planes of the neck as a result of gravity and movements of the muscles. Without delay a finger must be placed either extra- or intraorally to stop the tooth moving. A flap may then be raised to explore the tissue space when the tooth may be 'milked' out or removed as described for those under the periosteum. When the tooth is lying superficial to the mylohyoid, removal is better delayed to allow an extraoral approach, followed by a blunt dissection up to the tooth.

The unerupted upper third molar can be elevated distally into the soft tissue space behind the tuberosity of the maxilla to lie in the pterygomandibular space. This is explored through an incision made down the anterior border of the ascending ramus of the mandible.

Bone cavities

The roots of the maxillary second premolar, first, second and third molars and occasionally the first premolar are related to the maxillary sinus into which they can be displaced during extraction. Unerupted and supernumerary teeth may be related to the floor of the nose. Lower apices can be pushed into the inferior dental canal. In both jaws roots can be driven into pathological cavities such as cysts or abscesses. Where it is suspected that a root is lost in a bone cavity the operation is stopped and radiographs are taken in two planes at right angles to each other in an effort to localise the lost root or tooth.

Roots displaced into the inferior dental canal are removed by a transalveolar approach, care being taken not to damage the inferior dental nerve. They should not be left as they may give rise to infection or pressure symptoms of paraesthesia or anaesthesia. Roots pushed into the nose, if they lie under the mucous membrane, are usually easily recovered through the socket, or through the anterior nares if they are lying in the nasal cavity.

Oro-antral communication

The relationship of the apices of the maxillary premolar and molar teeth to the maxillary sinus is variable and depends on individual anatomy and the age of

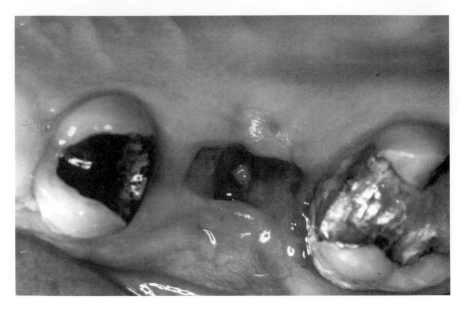

Fig. 10.1   Oro-antral fistula.

the patient as pneumatisation of the sinus continues throughout life. Often the antrum dips down between the roots of the molar teeth which virtually form part of the antral floor.

Occasionally the uncomplicated extraction of a tooth may fracture the thin floor of the sinus and cause an oro-antral communication. Apical infection can destroy the bone over the apex, bringing an apical granuloma into contact with antral lining which is then torn by the extraction of the tooth. Infection in the maxillary sinus may also predispose to the establishment of a fistula. More commonly the communication is produced by attempts to remove retained apices so that the antrum floor is perforated or the apex displaced into it (Fig. 10.1).

Signs and symptoms

The patient will complain of air passing from the nose into the mouth and this the operator will be able to see bubbling through the communication, particularly when the patient is asked to breathe out. Blood from the wound and mouthwashes used to rinse the mouth may pass through the sinus into the nose. A blunt probe passed very gently into the socket will be found to penetrate into the maxillary sinus. This last test should rarely be performed as it may create a communication. Established fistulae tend to reduce in diameter but the track from mouth to sinus frequently fails to heal spontaneously and becomes epithelialised. When this is large the patient complains that drinks pass from the mouth into the nose, that cigarettes are inhaled with difficulty, and that air passes into the mouth. As the hole shrinks it remains a pathway for infection,

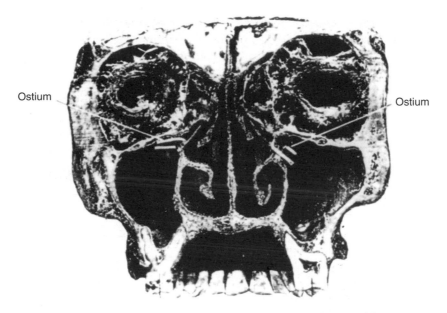

Ostium

Ostium

Fig. 10.2 Section through maxillary sinus. Ciliated mucosa allows rapid movement of mucus to give efficient drainage despite ostium being close to the root of the sinus.

but fails to provide adequate drainage for the sinus so that often the symptoms of acute sinusitis are superimposed on those of a fistula.

Treatment

Immediately the surgeon finds he has created a communication he should check that the tooth has been completely extracted. He should then gently remove all pieces of loose bone that might form sequestra. The buccal plate of alveolar bone is trimmed if a flap has been raised, but is otherwise left alone. Irrigation is best avoided. The mucous membrane over the socket is gently drawn together with simple interrupted sutures and every effort made to obtain a sound clot in the socket. *Under no circumstances should the socket be packed* with any material that will prevent healing. Thus ribbon guaze should be avoided at all costs. However a small piece of oxidised cellulose (Surgicel^R) to help to stabilise the clot may be of benefit in encouraging a seal. Impressions are taken and a splint constructed with a flange to cover and protect the socket. Before taking the impressions a sizeable piece of foil should be placed over the socket to protect the clot and to prevent the impression material being forced into the communication. The splint should be produced quickly as an emergency measure and, if possible, put in place the same day. Antibiotic therapy is commenced immediately and continued for some 5 days as a prophylactic measure whether or not there is a history of previous sinusitis. The patient is instructed that under no circumstances must he raise the pressure in his nose by blowing it until healing has taken place. Such energetic measures immediately applied will in most cases result in satisfactory healing by first intention.

Where the above measures fail and the fistula remains patent after 6 weeks, but there are no signs of maxillary sinus infection, a surgical repair should be undertaken without delay. This may be done under general anaesthesia as an in-patient or local anaesthesia as an out-patient, but always under an antibiotic cover started before operation. There are two commonly described methods, using a buccal or less commonly a palatal flap to cover the defect. In both cases the operation commences by excising the fistula cleanly and curetting out the tract from the socket. The deeper part of the fistula adjoining the antrum may be left undisturbed where there is no evidence of infection.

Buccal flap

This is the operation of choice. The flap is raised by making an incision along the buccal edge of the socket concerned and two vertical incisions from the cervical margins of the adjacent teeth obliquely up into the buccal sulcus. The flap is carefully raised well past the reflection. Normally this would not cover the socket because the periosteum is still attached, beyond the reflection, to maxillary bone. To overcome this the periosteum *only* is divided by a long horizontal incision made well *above* the line of reflection of the mucosa. It will then be found that the flap can be drawn down over the socket without tension (Fig. 10.3). Buttonholing of the buccal flap must obviously be avoided. The palatal mucoperiosteum is then trimmed back to a straight line so that

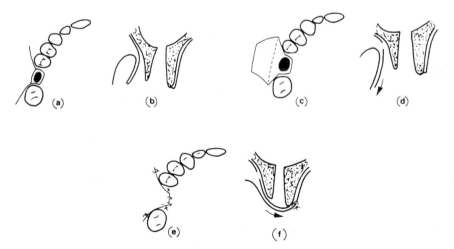

Fig. 10.3   Closure of oro-antral fistula using a buccal flap. (a) Show excision of fistula and buccal incision through mucoperiosteum. (b) Flap raised; note palatal mucosa trimmed back to expose ledge of palatal bone. (c) Dotted line shows incision through *periosteum only* above line of reflection of mucosa. (d) Mucosa extended once periosteum is divided. (e) and (f) Closure effected with buccal flap resting on palatal bone.

the line of closure will be supported by palatal bone. This margin is raised slightly to permit eversion of its edges when suturing. Haemorrhage is carefully arrested as a haematoma could prevent the flap taking, and closure is effected with mattress sutures. A splint may be worn over the wound to protect it. The only disadvantage of this operation is that it may reduce the depth of the buccal sulcus opposite the socket concerned but this is usually only temporary.

Palatal flap

The palatal flap is rarely used except in the repair of oro-nasal fistulae. It is a pedicle flap which derives its blood supply from the palatine artery and therefore has its base over the greater palatine foramen. It is raised by making an incision in the palate parallel to the cervical margins of the teeth but about 5 mm above them. This extends from the second molar to the lateral incisor and is then taken back almost down the midline of the palate. The flap is carefully raised with the periosteum to include the palatine artery. This must be preserved because if its function is impaired the flap will be deprived of its blood supply and die (Fig. 10.4). A second hazard to the artery occurs when the flap is rotated to cover the fistula, because if it is twisted too sharply, the blood supply may be cut off. Indeed this fact limits its use to the second premolar and first molar sockets. The buccal flap is trimmed back to a clean edge and, if possible, supported on bone though often loss of the buccal alveolar plate at the time of extraction makes this difficult to achieve. The flap is sutured into place with mattress sutures and the bone deficiency in the palate covered with a dressing (Fig. 10.4b). It has the advantage that the palatal flap is very thick and tough and is of sufficient length to cover the whole socket.

Infected maxillary sinus

Where the maxillary sinus is infected closure must not be attempted until this has settled.

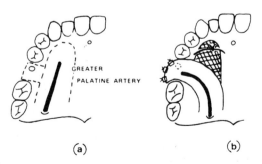

(a) (b)

Fig. 10.4 Oro-antral fistula. (a) design of palatal flap for closure of fistula showing the palatine artery in the flap and the excision of the fistula. (b) Closure showing rotation of the palatal flap and pack sutured over the area of bare bone.

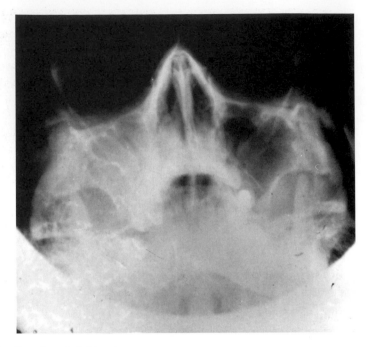

Fig. 10.5   Opacity of right antrum.

Acute sinusitis

In acute sinusitis the patient complains of pain together with a feeling of weight in the cheek on the affected side, especially on bending down. Discharge from the maxillary sinus is often described as 'catarrh' on that side, especially in the morning. Examination often shows the cheek over the infected sinus to be red, there is tenderness on pressure in the canine fossa and pus may be seen and smelled in the nostril. Transillumination and radiographs show opacity and, if pus is present, a fluid level (Fig. 10.5). Careful examination of the fistula will often show it to be inflamed or filled with granulations and discharging pus. The acute phase is treated with antibacterial drugs, and ephedrine nasal drops to reduce nasal congestion, and improve drainage through the ostium. Persistent symptoms of sinusitis may prevail after closure of a fistula. In these cases the opinon of an ENT surgeon is required. Intranasal antrostomy is rarely performed as this further disturbs the function of the ciliated epithelium of the sinus. Endoscopic sinus surgery may allow instrumentation to enable normal sinus function to resume.

Root in antrum

When a root is believed to have been pushed into the maxillary sinus the surgeon should first examine the socket carefully, and the adjacent sockets lest

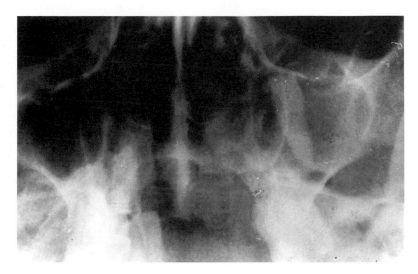

Fig. 10.6 Tooth in left antrum.

it should have been displaced there. He then considers whether the root is lying below the antral lining or has penetrated it to enter the sinus. Presence of an oro-antral communication is strong, but not conclusive, evidence that the root is in the antrum. Radiographs, apical intraoral and oblique occlusal films are required (Fig. 10.6). It is usual to take a second set after shaking the head to see if the root has moved, if it has it is probably lying free in the sinus cavity. The root if fixed may be jammed under the lining, though this is not certain as it can be lying in the antrum anchored by a blood clot.

Where the root is believed to be lying under the lining it may be removed through a transalveolar approach, care being taken not to damage the antral lining. This is better than through an extranasal antrostomy as it is often very difficult to locate roots under the lining when looking into the antrum.

Roots which are lying in the antral cavity and remain in close relation to the socket are best removed through a transalveolar approach. Where the root is grossly displaced the Caldwell–Luc extranasal antrostomy is preferable. For this latter operation the patient is admitted to hospital and, under general anaesthesia and an antibiotic cover, an incision is made in the mucous membrane of the canine fossa above its reflection into the cheek. A flap is reflected to expose the anterior wall of the antrum. The infraorbital nerve must not be damaged, particularly by stretching when retracting the flap during the operation. With chisels or burs a round hole about 1.5 cm in diameter is cut through the thin anterior wall, above the roots of the teeth and near to the lateral wall of the nose. All spicules of loose bone are carefully removed and the interior inspected using a headlamp. Suction should be used very carefully to avoid damaging the delicate lining. The root is lifted out with sinus forceps and, if infection is present, drainage is provided by a tube drain inserted through the buccal incision. The mouth wound is then closed.

Damage to soft tissues

The chief cause of damage to soft tissues is carelessness by the operator. The gingivae can be torn by misapplication of dental forceps, pulling on teeth to which gingival margins are still attached instead of dissecting them free, and by attempting the removal of roots without adequate access. When extracting upper teeth the lower lip can be trapped between the forceps and the lower teeth.

The cheek, tongue, floor of mouth and palate can be damaged by instruments which slip because they are not properly supported. This applies particularly to elevators, burs and discs. A disc guard must always be used. Burns are caused by hot instruments from the steriliser, overheating of burs or handpieces, and antiseptic solutions.

Nerves

The inferior dental nerve can be damaged during the extraction of buried teeth or retained roots. Its relationship to the third molar has been discussed (Chapter 9). When a flap is raised for operations in the lower premolar area the mental nerve should be identified and preserved. Stretching of nerves when retracting flaps can produce paraesthesia which may be very painful and of long duration and this can occur with the mental and infraorbital nerves. The lingual nerve where it lies in the lingual mucoperiosteum of the mandible opposite the third molar can be damaged when this tooth is being extracted.

Fracture of alveolar and basal bone

The buccal and lingual alveolar plates

These can be fractured during the extraction of teeth, particularly if as a result of chronic periodontal disease the tooth is ankylosed or exostosed to the socket wall. The buccal plate in the molar region is most frequently involved but is usually firmly attached to periosteum which provides it with a satisfactory blood supply. This bone can be retained if it is repositioned by gently compressing the socket between finger and thumb after completing the extractions.

Loose fragments not attached to periosteum must be removed lest they form sequestra, suppurate and delay healing.

Occasionally extraction of a tooth causes a horizontal fracture of the alveolus which may carry other teeth. This occurs classically in the maxilla during an attempted extraction of single standing upper molars, especially the third molar, and may cause fracture of the tuberosity. This will be felt during the extraction by the movement of bone rather than the tooth and a radiograph should be taken to confirm the presence of a fracture. Where the portion of bone attached to the tooth is small, bone and tooth should be dissected out by blunt dissection through a buccal flap, taking every precaution to prevent tearing of the mucous membrane. The antrum is frequently opened following this manoeuvre, but if the flaps are healthy it can be closed satisfactorily. The surgeon may wish to retain a large piece of bone or one with other teeth, not for extraction, attached to it. It is very difficult to hold the bone still and complete the planned extraction. So long as any pain from the tooth can be alleviated the fragment can be splinted for a month until it is firm. The tooth may then be extracted by freeing it from the bone with burs and gently prising it out with elevators. This procedure is seldom justified unless sound teeth in occlusion are to be saved.

Basal bone

The predisposing causes of fracture of the body of the mandible are general bone diseases (osteogenesis imperfecta, osteopetrosis), weakened bone owing to age, osteomyelitis, cysts, tumours, teeth with large or misplaced roots and buried teeth. The immediate cause is misapplication of instruments or the use of undue force, particularly with elevators. As soon as the operator realises that a fracture has occurred he should complete the operation if this can be done without causing further damage. Radiographs must be taken to confirm the position and extent of the injury, and the patient referred immediately for treatment by reduction and fixation (Chapter 14).

Dislocation of the temporomandibular joint

This occurs most frequently following the extraction of lower teeth under general anaesthesia but may happen even under local anaesthesia in those patients who have a lax capsule and weak supporting muscles.

Dislocation may be prevented by supporting the mandible firmly and never exerting more force in the primary downward movement than can be opposed by the supporting hand. During extractions under local anaesthesia a prop placed on the opposite side of the mouth gives the patient something to bite on and thereby support his jaw.

At the close of operations under general anaesthesia the jaws should be brought together with the teeth in occlusion at the time the prop and pack are removed from the mouth. The jaw, if dislocated, may be reduced before the patient returns to full consciousness (Chapter 17).

Post-extraction

Haemorrhage

Prolonged haemorrhage is a common complication following extraction of teeth and occurs as primary (Chapter 7), reactionary and secondary haemorrhage.

The most important aspect of treatment is prevention. The systemic causes have been discussed in Chapter 3, but local factors are more often responsible for post-operative haemorrhage. These include infection, excessive trauma and local vascular lesions.

Infections include gingival conditions, which should be treated by scaling and instructions in oral hygiene. To be effective, scaling should be completed a week before operation and mouth-brushing conscientiously undertaken by the patient. This preparation should be done for all but emergency extractions, and the dental surgeon must stress the importance of a clean mouth as many patients tend to neglect oral hygiene on the ground that they are about to lose their remaining teeth. Where there is an apical or pericoronal condition the use of antibiotics may be indicated, not only to prevent a flare up but to protect the blood clot from destruction by bacteria.

Reactionary haemorrhage

Reactionary haemorrhage occurs within 48 hours of the operation or accident when a local rise in blood pressure may force open divided vessels insecurely sealed by natural or artificial means. It is common in patients recovering from shock and in those treated under local anaesthesia when the effect of the vasoconstrictor wears off. It is arrested by one of the methods described below and, for excited patients, by administration of a sedative.

Secondary haemorrhage

The cause of secondary haemorrhage is infection which destroys the blood clot or may ulcerate a vessel wall. It starts about 7 days after operation, usually with a mild ooze which is a serious symptom in wounds near major vessels because, if the vessel is not found and ligated, a massive haemorrhage may ensue. In the more mild capillary form such as from a tooth socket it will be more troublesome than dangerous. Bleeding is arrested by local measures and antibacterial drugs are prescribed to combat the infection.

Treatment

A practitioner who is called to a post-extraction haemorrhage should first take from the patient, or a relative, a *rapid* history which must include the number of teeth extracted, the duration of bleeding (the volume of the loss is unreliable as it is invariably diluted by saliva), and whether there has been any similar previous occurrence or known blood dyscrasia. The patient's general condition is then rapidly assessed and, if he appears shocked and ill, arrangements must be made at once for transfer to hospital. Meanwhile the dental surgeon will apply local measures to arrest the bleeding.

It is never a waste of time to clean the patient, for much of the distress and fear associated with bleeding is due to the sight of blood on the face, sheets and clothes. The mouth is then examined in a good light with adequate suction apparatus, if available. The latter should only be used to remove blood from the floor of the mouth and not be applied to the sockets since aspiration will disturb stable blood clots and encourage further bleeding. Pressure is then applied by placing a finger on each side of the alveolus to find the bleeding point. If this is successful in arresting the haemorrhage it indicates bleeding from soft tissues, and sutures may be placed across the socket. Where pressure fails to arrest the haemorrhage, bleeding is from the bony socket and an oxidised cellulose pack may be placed in the socket. When local measures have controlled the bleeding, the patient's general condition should be more accurately assessed by recording his pulse and blood pressure. He should receive supportive treatment including warmth, administration of fluids by mouth, and drugs to relieve anxiety and pain.

Surgical emphysema

Surgical emphysema is a collection of air which has been forced into the tissue spaces through the extraction wound and forms a swelling which characteristically crackles on palpation. It results from increased air pressure in the mouth from using an air spray, or blowing a trumpet or a balloon. Surgical emphysema seldom gives rise to discomfort, but settles without treatment as the air is slowly absorbed.

Delayed healing and infection

Normally a tooth socket heals by second intention, the blood clot becoming organised as capillaries and fibroblasts grow into it from the bony or soft tissue periphery. The blood clot may fail to form if there is little bleeding owing to sclerosis of the bone forming the tooth socket, the action of the vasoconstrictor present in the local anaesthetic solution, or packing of the socket to arrest haemorrhage. Infection may rapidly supervene if the extracted tooth was septic or contamination takes place from the mouth. Even where a satisfactory clot does form, this can be destroyed by bacteria either present in the socket or introduced by imperfectly sterilised instruments. Lacerated or bruised tissues, loose pieces of bone or retained tooth fragments also favour secondary infection.

Early loss of the blood clot produces an acutely painful condition in around 5% of normal extractions. The socket contains either remnants of the blood clot or food debris. The aetiology of this condition is unclear although infection has been mooted. The blood clot fails to organise and healing is subsequently delayed on account of which the socket may become secondarily infected. A decrease in blood supply to the healing socket may be one of the factors and a higher incidence has been seen following the use of local anaesthetic containing adrenaline. Smoking also seems to increase the chance of developing dry socket. Treatment is aimed at protecting the socket during the production of granulation tissue over the exposed socket walls. Packing materials that contain some analgesic and sedative properties together with an antiseptic are used once the socket has been irrigated with warm saline to remove any debris. Various materials are available such as Alvogyl[R], an iodoform dressing that does not need to be removed, and bismuth, iodoform and paraffin paste (BIPP) on ribbon gauze. This dressing may have to be removed and replaced on occasions until the socket has epithelialised after about 3 weeks.

Post-extraction infection may take another form in which exuberant granulations and a discharge of pus localised to the socket appear a week or so after the extraction. Frequently bone sequestra are the cause and when they are removed healing takes place rapidly. This condition is relatively painless and the granulations make packing difficult. Treatment is first by hot mouth baths but, if these fail to settle the socket, radiographs are necessary to confirm the local nature of the infection. The socket is then opened up, sequestra and granulations removed and the cavity packed open. Forceful curettage is contraindicated as it may spread the infection.

Infected sockets are a serious condition which if neglected may progress to osteomyelitis or to a severe cellulitis of the face and neck (Chapter 12).

Damage to other organs

Faulty or careless handling of instruments may result in damage to other organs. Under general anaesthesia the eyes, if not suitably protected, can be damaged by caustic fluids, instruments and the operator's fingers.

Pain

Post-extraction pain may result from incomplete extraction of the tooth, laceration of the soft tissues, exposed bone, infected sockets or damage to adjacent nerves. Treatment is by eliminating the cause and symptomatic by prescribing analgesic drugs.

Swelling

Swelling or oedema following surgery is part of the inflammatory reaction to surgical interference. It is increased by a poor surgical technique, particularly rough handling of the tissues, pulling on flaps to gain access and inadequate drainage. There is also a wide individual variation in the response to trauma which does not seem to be related to any of these factors.

Trismus

Trismus may occur as the result of oedema and swelling, in which case opening improves as the swelling resolves. Damage to the temporomandibular joint due to excessive downward pressure or to keeping the patient's mouth open wide for a long period may lead to a more chronic, painful condition with symptoms of the pain dysfunction syndrome (Chapter 17). The injection for the inferior dental nerve block may cause a painless trismus without swelling which has variously been ascribed to trauma to the medial pterygoid muscle causing spasm, or to penetration of a small blood vessel and formation of a haematoma. As the haematoma organises so the trismus becomes apparent, often starting 2–3 days after the injection. It will recover with time, usually 6 weeks, but may be improved more quickly by gently opening the mouth under a general anaesthetic.

Broken instruments

All instruments should be carefully examined after use and any that are defective immediately discarded or sent for repair. Should one break, a search is made at once for the fragment and if it is not recovered radiographs are taken to locate it. If the instrument is sterile and the piece small, such as the point of a suture needle or a tiny portion of a dental bur, this may be left and the patient informed (Fig. 10.7).

Broken local anaesthetic needles occur chiefly when giving an inferior dental nerve block. The needle should never be inserted up to the hub but one-third of its length must be kept clear of the tissues. A pair of artery forceps should

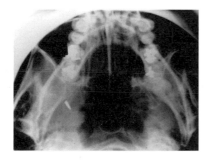

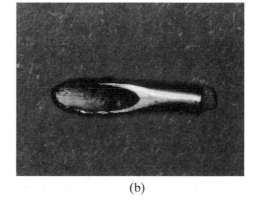

(a) (b)

Fig. 10.7 Broken instrument: (a) a fragment can be seen in the lingual tissues adjacent to the third molar socket; (b) the retrieved fragment: the end of an elevator which fractured during the removal of the lower third molar. The patient suffered temporary loss of sensation in the lingual nerve.

always be close at hand to grasp the fragment immediately before it disappears if the patient moves or swallows.

Removal of broken needles from the pterygomandibular space is a difficult operation. First the needle must be localised by taking radiographs in two planes (lateral oblique and posterior anterior views of the mandible), preferably with a second needle in position to serve as a marker. At operation, performed under endotracheal anaesthesia, a vertical incision is made parallel to the anterior border of the ascending ramus, blunt dissection is performed down to the marker and a search is made in the vicinity for the broken needle. A metallic foreign body detector can be of great assistance.

Mishaps

The patient or a relative should always be warned beforehand if any serious difficulty or complication is envisaged and this should be entered on the consent form signed by the patient.

When a mishap has occurred it is important to keep quite calm and not become emotionally involved. The patient is often upset, aggressive and vociferous, and the surgeon must not allow himself to get caught up in this mood. He may, and indeed should, state what has happened quite factually without making any comment or explanation which might imply liability. If the patient is nervous it is best to tell a sensible relative or, failing that, the patient's medical or dental practitioner. In any serious accident, such as a fracture of the jaw or a root in antrum, it is very wise to hand the case over to a colleague, preferably a specialist, as thereafter the responsibility is shared. It is also wise when treating a mishap to limit the immediate care to putting it right, and not to attempt the completion of all the surgery planned, as a new disaster may occur elsewhere in the mouth.

In any case of doubt the practitioners' protection society should be informed at the earliest possible time and asked for advice and guidance, which they will willingly give.

Further reading

McGowan, D.A., Baxter, P.W. & Jones, J. (1993) *The Maxillary Sinus and its Dental Implications.* Wright, Oxford.

Mulcahy, L., Rosenthal, M.M. & Lloyd-Bostock, S.M. (1998) *Medical Mishaps: pieces of the puzzle.* Open University Press, Buckingham.

Robinson, P.P. (1988) Observations on the recovery of sensation following inferior alveolar nerve injuries. *British Journal of Oral and Maxillofacial Surgery*, **26**, 177.

Chapter 11
Preparation of the Mouth for Dentures

- Preservation of alveolar bone
- Surgical preparation at time of extraction
- Surgical preparation of the edentulous mouth
- Increasing the size of the alveolar ridge
- Ridge augmentation
- Implants

The surgical preparation of the mouth for dentures begins at the time the first permanent tooth is extracted. At this and all subsequent operations the oral surgeon must try to leave a satisfactory base to support a prosthesis and he should consider the form the denture-bearing tissues will present when healing and resorption of bone is complete. Edentulous patients should not be subjected to surgery to improve the stability, comfort or aesthetic appearance of their dentures without the opinion of a specialist prosthetist.

Ideally, treatment for those undergoing clearances or surgical preparation for dentures should be planned jointly. This assists the surgeon and enables the prosthetist to make valuable pre-operative records of the occlusion and of the tooth form and shade. Further, to assist denture retention certain teeth may be selected for conservation rather than extraction. Consideration should be given to retaining roots and provision of overdentures to maintain alveolar bone height. In general dental practice, surgeon and prosthetist are the same person, offering an unrivalled opportunity for treatment planning and for long-term evaluation of the results of surgery. The oral surgeon will learn much from reviewing his patients over several years and discussing, with the dental surgeon who constructs the denture, any problems that occur.

Preservation of alveolar bone

It should always be borne in mind that alveolar bone is precious and once lost cannot be replaced. This tissue, possibly more than any other, suffers from instrument mismanagement. A conservative approach and a careful surgical technique will help to reduce prosthetic difficulties later.

During extractions the alveolar bone may be damaged or fractured by the use of excessive force or worse, by the inclusion of the socket wall within the forcep blades. The commonest site of alveolar fracture is the buccal plate opposite the upper molars. This, if still attached to periosteum, may be preserved and pressed back into place, but if detached from its blood supply it should be removed to avoid sequestration and delayed healing. Fracture and loss of the maxillary tuberosity may interfere with retention of the upper denture by making the peripheral seal at this point inadequate.

The bone of the edentulous jaws in the elderly is often dense and brittle whilst resorption of the alveolar ridge has made it less strong. Under such conditions the extraction of buried teeth and roots is difficult. Those that are symptomless need not be extracted if they are covered by bone and are unlikely to come to the surface during the life of the denture. Those lying superficially or associated with secondary disease such as cysts or granulomas should be removed. Roots and teeth must be accurately localised and tooth division practised to reduce the amount of bone removed. This is confined as far as possible to the buccal aspect and osteoplastic flaps are used to preserve the ridge where teeth are lying in it (Chapter 9).

The use of blunt burs or failure to provide irrigation with a continuous stream of saline can cause overheating with subsequent necrosis of bone.

Surgical preparation at the time of extraction of teeth

The operation is carefully planned to include the removal of buried teeth roots, or other lesions. Any necessary adjustments to the alveolar bone are marked on plaster models and, because this bone can never be replaced, every effort is made to reduce cutting or smoothing to a minimum. Difficult extractions are best completed through a planned transalveolar approach to avoid accidental alveolar fractures which lead to widespread trimming to produce an acceptable ridge. For multirooted teeth, particularly upper molars, division of the roots so that each is removed separately may conserve alveolar bone. Access to deeply buried roots or teeth can often be made through the lateral aspect of the alveolus, to leave the ridge intact. In all such operations bone cutting should be limited to one side, leaving the lingual or palatal plate and its mucoperiosteum untouched. Alveolectomy at the time of extraction requires careful consideration as, even after radical surgical reduction, some natural resorption takes place and it is impossible to tell how extensive this will be. Generally it is advisable to do the minimum at the time of extraction and wait for at least three months to reconsider the situation when healing and natural remodelling has taken place. A conservative approach is important where periodontal disease has already caused appreciable bone loss.

There are certain indications for minor surgery at the time of the extractions:

(1) Jagged or irregular alveolar margins and septal bone, which are treated by dividing the buccal interdental papillae from the lingual along the ridge and exposing the bony edges of the sockets just enough to smooth the bone with a bur or file, after which the mucosa is closed over the ridge.
(2) Minor local deformities, such as fibrous bands, bulbous tuberosities, and undercuts may be removed.
(3) The premaxilla may need reduction in cases of superior protrusion.

Surgery for immediate restoration dentures

Where a complete immediate denture is to be provided the posterior teeth are first extracted. Sufficient teeth are left in the premolar region to maintain the vertical dimension of the occlusion while the sockets are healing. Three months later the rest of the teeth are removed. When, owing to the tightness of the lip, an anterior flange cannot be worn an open-faced denture with the anterior teeth socketed into the alveolus is provided as a temporary measure until natural resorption has taken place. In certain cases, however, it is obvious that some reduction is necessary at the time the teeth are extracted.

Where the patient must be admitted to hospital the less satisfactory procedure of fitting a full mouth immediate restoration denture can be performed.

Alveolectomy for pre-maxillary protrusion

The prosthetist and the surgeon who is to do the operation should examine the patient and prepare the models for the dentures. Articulated models in duplicate and panoramic radiographs are required. On one model the teeth on one side only are removed and the plaster trimmed back to a satisfactory depth, which must not be more than half the diameter of the sockets, and teeth are set up to occlude with the lower dentition to estimate the improvement achieved. Frequently it will be necessary to reduce the height of the alveolus to give sufficient space to fit artificial teeth. When one half of the model is prepared the untouched half provides a useful comparative record of the original state. The second model is then trimmed to the same amount but on both sides and used to process the dentures. A thin template in clear acrylic, which must be quite transparent, is prepared on a duplicate of this model.

At operation an incision is made round the necks of the teeth with two short vertical extensions just beyond the standing teeth at each end. The teeth are then extracted and the flap reflected. Using rongeurs or a large rosehead bur, the ridge is cut to the size planned and left smooth with no sharp projections from the interradicular septa. The soft tissues are then replaced and the transparent template pressed firmly over them. High spots show as blanched areas of mucous membrane. These need further reduction before final smoothing is completed with a bone file.

Surgical preparation of the edentulous mouth

Before prosthetic surgery the edentulous patient must have a clinical examination and panoramic radiographs to avoid missing conditions such as buried roots or residual cysts. The surgery requires skill and patience as the soft tissues can be difficult to manipulate and slow to heal owing to scarring following repeated ulceration or to friability caused by the atrophic changes of age. The operation must leave minimal scarring so placed that it receives the least pressure from the dentures.

Bony irregularities

Torus

A large palatal torus is usually acceptable if smooth but when nodular or irregular in shape may need to be removed. Tori, often bilateral, are sometimes found on the lingual aspect of the mandible in the premolar region and can cause pain or difficulty when a full denture is worn. The torus palatinus is excised through a Y-shaped midline sagittal incision and the bony prominence removed with burs or chisels. A full denture lined with a periodontal dressing is immediately fitted to hold the flap in place and prevent formation of a haematoma (Fig. 11.1).

Alveolar ridges

These should be of substantial size, as the greater their surface area the better is the denture retained and the more evenly are masticatory pressures distributed. In grossly resorbed ridges the dentures are loose as there is nothing to resist horizontal displacement. This may be aggravated by failure of the peripheral seal due to the lifting action of certain muscles (buccinator, mylohyoid and genioglossus), the attachments of which become level with the alveolar crest. In the mandible the mental foramen can open on the crest of the ridge and

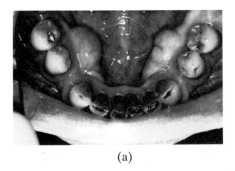
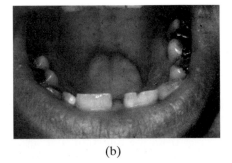

(a) (b)

Fig. 11.1 Tori: (a) mandibular tori would cause problems when denture is worn; (b) Palatal torus.

cause pain from pressure of the denture. Occasionally ridges may be too high making it difficult to fit dentures without over opening the vertical dimension.

Undercut ridges are unfavourable if the flange has to be built out from the alveolus to avoid them as this reduces the peripheral seal. However, certain undercuts may be retained to assist retention providing the problem of fitting the denture round them can be overcome.

Even when considerable resorption of the edentulous ridge has taken place it may be irregular. This can follow tooth extraction where the expanded buccal plate has not been adequately compressed or when it fractures and jagged edges are left. These cause pain when the mucosa is compressed between the sharp bone and the denture during chewing.

Alveolectomy

This is the operation used to smooth irregular ridges and remove undercuts. Radiographs must be studied to determine the extent of the antrum and the position of the mental nerve. Plaster casts of the ridges are used to assist planning so that the procedure is completed with the least destruction of alveolar bone.

A horizontal incision is made on the buccal aspect of the alveolus through fixed mucoperiosteum just short of non-keratinised mucosa so that this is not disturbed by the operation. Two vertical incisions are taken over the crest of the alveolus and on to the lingual or palatal mucosa. The flap is reflected to expose the alveolar crest (Fig. 11.2). The bone may be trimmed with a large rosehead bur or rongeurs and smoothed with a bone file. The operator then replaces the flap and runs his finger over the ridge to check it is smooth. The wound is thoroughly irrigated with saline and if much reduction has taken place the flap is trimmed conservatively. The wound is closed without tension on the mucoperiosteum.

Feather edge ridge

This condition occurs in the lower anterior region beneath a full lower denture. The patient complains of inability to wear the denture for more than one or

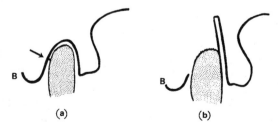

(a)   (b)

Fig. 11.2 Alveolectomy. B indicates buccal aspect of ridge. (a) Arrow shows level of buccal horizontal incision above the reflection. (b) Flap raised from buccal to lingual to expose alveolar ridge without interference with attachment of mucoperiosteum at the buccal or lingual reflection.

two hours owing to soreness. The ridge is usually very narrow and covered with thin atrophic mucosa which is inflamed and tender to palpation. Radiographs show an uneven resorbed ridge which has no cortical plate but a feathered appearance due to spicules of bone standing vertically.

Surgery should be considered only when all prosthetic techniques to reduce the load (selective compression impressions, narrow teeth and resilient linings) have failed.

Treatment

Surgical treatment has not proved to be very effective. Alveolectomy may be performed but when this is limited to smoothing the knife-edge ridge relief is usually only temporary. Even when the ridge is drastically reduced, so that the denture virtually rests on basal bone, the symptoms often persist. In view of this, attention has been directed to the mucosa. Though histological examination has shown scant changes in this, better results have been obtained by excising the mucoperiosteum over the ridge and replacing it with a free mucoperiosteal graft taken from the maxillary ridge or palate.

Genial tubercles

These sometimes become prominent in the floor of the mouth owing to alveolar recession. They are best left, as genioglossus is attached to them. Occasionally, the upper part of a prominent genial tubercule may require excision to facilitate denture wearing.

Mylohyoid ridge removal

Where the mandibular alveolus has undergone gross resorption the mylohyoid ridge, if sharp, may be a source of pain under the lower denture. Its removal, by cutting off the attachment of the mylohyoid muscle, does deepen the lingual sulcus of the mandible and may assist denture retention when the muscle attachment is level with the alveolar crest.

An incision is made along the alveolar crest and reflected lingually to expose the mylohyoid muscle which is detached from the bone. The prominent bony mylohyoid ridge is then separated from the mandible with burs. Bleeding is meticulously arrested and the incision closed. This procedure may be carried out in combination with sulcus deepening in the anterior mandible (see later in this chapter).

Soft tissue irregularities

Flabby ridges

Ideally the alveolar mucosa should be firm and closely adherent to the ridge, but after the extraction of teeth for periodontal disease hyperplastic tissue may remain to form a flabby ridge. More often such ridges are found in the anterior region of the maxilla when a full upper denture is opposed only by the natural lower anterior teeth. The excessive pressure causes resorption of the maxillary bone leaving a thick mobile fibrous ridge offering an unstable support for the denture. However, as this is better than the completely flat surface often left by surgery, the prosthetist prefers to manage this problem with special impression techniques and denture design. An alternative approach is to augment the underlying bone using a bone substitute material to provide support for the soft tissue. If there is sufficient bone depth consideration should be given to the use of implants.

Reduction of tuberosities

Large maxillary tuberosities with deep sulci assist denture retention but if too large they encroach on the space available for dentures. Many have appreciable bony undercuts on their buccal aspect which, if unilateral, can be used to improve denture stability but when present bilaterally prevent a satisfactory fit. Radiographs before surgery are necessary to identify unerupted upper third molars, to establish the relationship between soft tissue and alveolar bone and to determine the extent of the maxillary antrum.

Treatment

A fibrous tuberosity may be reduced by making palatal and buccal incisions down to bone to excise an ellipse of mucous membrane, fibrous tissue and periosteum from the crest of the ridge. To facilitate closure the incisions are carried forward to meet in the first molar region. The raw edges are then undermined and the underlying fibrous tissue removed to produce a reduction in the height of the ridge and to allow satisfactory closure (Fig. 11.3). The space between upper and lower ridges is checked to be satisfactory before the wound is sutured.

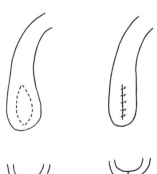

Fig. 11.3 Reduction of the tuberosity. (a) Above: Elliptical incision over tuberosity. Below: Cross-section of excision showing deep portion secondarily excised (shaded) to allow flaps to be apposed on bone without tension. (b) Closure.

Where only the bone is to be reduced in height or a buccal undercut removed the approach is made through an alveolectomy flap. Care is required not to perforate the antral lining when cutting bone in this region. Usually both bone and soft tissue are to be reduced and the elliptical incision is used to expose the ridge by reflecting the edges of the wound. Buccal undercuts in this area are often found high above the crest making necessary a vertical incision at the anterior buccal edge of the ellipse.

Fraenectomy

A fraenum is a musculo-fibrous band attached to the alveolus and inserted into the muscles of the face. The most important of these are the labial fraena in the mid-line of the upper and lower jaw, the buccal fraena in the premolar region and the lingual fraenum of the mandible. During movements of the facial muscles they lift the dentures and so break the peripheral seal. The denture can usually be relieved round them but where the ridges have resorbed this may greatly reduce the possible depth of the flange and even weaken the denture, making surgery by excision necessary.

Treatment

The maxillary labial fraenum is excised as follows. First the extent of its attachment to the maxilla is found by drawing the upper lip forward to put the fraenum on tension. This causes the base to blanch and it is frequently seen to extend palatally into the incisive papilla. The whole length of the fraenum and the mucosa over it is removed but the periosteum is left intact. A diamond-shaped incision is made round the margins of the band sufficiently deep to allow it to be dissected out and for the portion in the lip to the superficially excised (Fig. 11.4). The mucosa is undermined before suturing. The effect of suturing the lateral edges of the diamond-shaped incision together is to lengthen the wound and mobilise the soft tissues. This allows a greater depth of sulcus to be achieved.

Fraena may be lengthened by making a *horizontal* incision across the middle of the band which passes through the *whole depth* of the fibrous tissue it contains. The mucosal edges are undermined and the incision is sutured *vertically* (Figs 11.4 and 11.5).

Denture irritation hyperplasia

This is a fibroepithelial overgrowth in response to chronic trauma. The cause is an overextended denture flange which transmits the masticatory forces to the soft tissues. This situation often occurs following resorption of the ridges (Fig. 11.6).

The denture hyperplasia may present as one fold or a series of folds like the leaves of a book, which lie in the buccal sulcus either between the alveolus and the denture or along the periphery of the flange. (Fig. 11.6)

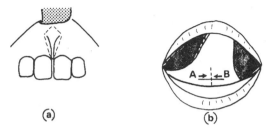

Fig. 11.4 Fraena. (a) Incision for excision of labial fraenum. (b) Lingual fraenum lengthened by making a horizontal incison A–B and suturing it vertically.

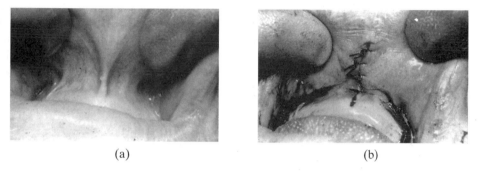

(a) (b)

Fig. 11.5 Frenectomy: (a) tight labial frenum; (b) following frenectomy.

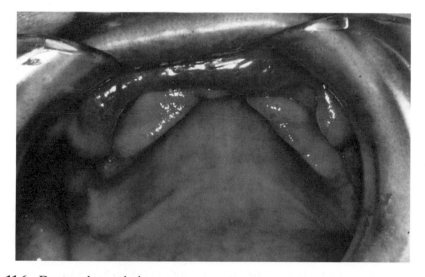

Fig. 11.6 Denture hyperplasia.

Treatment

First the irritation is removed by leaving out the denture or easing back the flange. The patient is reviewed after one month and if satisfactory recession has not taken place, it should be excised.

A single hyperplastic fold is removed by grasping it between toothed forceps and cutting through its base. The edges of the wound are then undermined and sutured without altering the depth of the buccal sulcus. Large multi-leaved hyperplasias require excision, and the raw area covered with a split thickness skin graft or a mucosal graft from the cheek or palate. This may be combined with sulcus deepening if necessary.

Cryosurgery has been used and leaves a satisfactory sulcus, but has the disadvantage that no tissue is obtained for biopsy and that the area can be very sore and swollen after operation. An alternative is to excise the hyperplastic tissue using the CO_2 laser. Here the wound is left open and re-epithelialises with minimal contraction or scarring.

Papillary hyperplasia

This presents as multiple small elevations of fibroepithelial hyperplasia, often associated with chronic candidiasis. Treatment may be with antifungal agents and where indicated surgery. Where the lesion is extensive or there is doubt about its benign nature the area is excised. In less severe cases the small hyperplasias can be removed by crysosurgery or by shaving off the elevations using rotary abrasives.

Increasing the size of the alveolar ridge

There are two aspects to surgically increasing the denture bearing area:

- Sulcus deepening
- Ridge augmentation

Sulcus deepening

The size of the denture-bearing area can be increased by deepening the sulci providing there is adequate underlying bone. That this is difficult to do satisfactorily is proved by the number of operations designed to this end, of which only a few are described here. Deepening of the buccal sulcus in the maxilla is seldom necessary as the palate provides a large denture-bearing area. Retention and support for the lower denture would often benefit from deepening of the sulci particularly where muscle attachments have come to lie near the crest of the ridge. Anteriorly the mentalis muscle, laterally the buccinator muscle, and lingually the mylohyoid muscle are involved. To deepen the sulci effectively these muscles must be detached from the mandible and the mucosa made to heal with a new reflection at a lower level. This last is the most difficult part of the operation. It is complicated by the presence of the mental nerve which must be located and preserved from accidental damage.

The procedures available can be considered in four groups.

The mucosa is advanced to line both sides of an extended sulcus (submucosal vestibuloplasty)

An example of this group is Obwegeser's operation. This attempts to divide the muscle attachments and deepen the buccal sulcus without making a flap or leaving raw areas. The procedure is usually performed in the maxilla. Two vertical incisions 1 cm long are made in the buccal sulcus of the canine regions or a single incision in the mid-line. Scissors or a scalpel are then passed between mucosa and periosteum. The muscle attachments on the buccal aspect are cut, as far back and upwards as possible, to free the mucosa. This is drawn up and the sulcus maintained by using a denture lined with gutta percha. One or two bone screws in the palate retain the denture for 2 weeks. Obwegeser's operation has the disadvantage that it is performed blind and if bleeding occurs the new sulcus may be obliterated.

Skin is transplanted to line both sides of an extended sulcus (buccal inlay)

In this operation a pouch is made in the mandibular buccal sulcus which is lined with a split-thickness skin graft from the patient's arm or thigh. An incision is made in the mandibular labial sulcus and a pouch dissected to the required size. This must leave the periosteum intact and attached to bone. An acrylic splint with a gutta percha mould, larger than will eventually be required, is made. Where the skin graft and mucous membrane meet, the mould is grooved so that on healing the ring scar contracts into the groove. The mould is chilled and the skin graft attached to it with the raw surface outwards. This is then placed in the pouch and the splint secured to the mandible with circumferential wires for two weeks.

Skin is transplanted to line one side of an extended sulcus (lower labial vestibuloplasty)

An incision is made along the mandibular alveolar crest from canine to canine. The incision goes through the mucosa but *not* through the mentalis muscle or the periosteum. The mucosal flap is dissected off periosteum and muscles. Care must be taken not to tear the mucosa. Dissection is continued past the reflection, just short of the inner margin of the lip. The mentalis muscle is then divided with a scapel close to the periosteum, which is left undisturbed. The muscle will retract into the deeper tissues. The mucosal flap is repositioned to cover the labial side of the new sulcus and held in position by sutures through the periosteum. A split-thickness skin graft is placed against the raw area of the periosteum with a gutta percha mould on an acrylic splint. In this way, the labial aspect of the new sulcus is lined with mucosa, and the periosteum with the skin graft.

Lowering of floor of mouth and vestibuloplasty

This operation, described by Obwegeser, combines a buccal vestibuloplasty and skin graft with a vestibuloplasty on the lingual aspect of the ridge which heals by secondary epithelialisation. The mucosal flaps on the buccal and lingual sides are held down in the depths of the new sulci by sutures passing under the mandible.

In the vestibuloplasty procedures, the splint or modified denture must be maintained in place for 2–3 weeks to allow initial healing. During this period, a high standard of oral hygiene is vital. Following removal of the splint, there is a marked tendency for the sulcus to contract. To reduce this, the denture must be modified to extend into the full depth of the sulcus and be worn continuously for several weeks.

Ridge augmentation

The height or breadth of the ridge can be increased by the introduction of material under the mucoperiosteum. This may be achieved by:

- Bone grafting
- Onlay bone grafting
- Interpositional bone grafting
- Sinus lift procedures
- Bone substitutes

Bone grafting

All these techniques have the disadvantage of a second surgical site for the harvesting of bone. This increases the morbidity of the procedure in the elderly patient. Significant resorption of the graft has been reported and loading of the area is delayed for up to 6 months.

Areas with little bone depth may require bone grafting before the provision of implants.

Onlay bone grafting

Autogenous bone from iliac crest or rib may be laid on the denture-bearing surface of the ridge under the mucoperiosteum. This is most often used in the mandible. The graft may be secured with wires or titanium bone screws. Osseointegrated implants may be placed at the time of grafting or after the graft has stabilised at around 6 months.

Interpositional bone grafting

The alveolar ridge is osteotomised horizontally to allow the placement of a block of bone between the basal bone and the alveolus. This is usually performed in the anterior region of the mandible to avoid damage to the mental nerve.

Sinus lift procedure

This is performed to increase bone depth prior to implant insertion in the posterior maxilla. The antral lining is exposed through a Caldwell-Luc approach and carefully dissected from the underlying bone. Bone graft is then placed to lift the sinus lining and effectively increase the depth of alveolar bone. As this does not affect the denture-bearing area directly, dentures can continue to be worn until implant placement has been completed.

Bone substitutes

Bone substitutes have the advantage of avoiding a second surgical site for harvesting of bone. However, the poor long term success due to migration of the implanted material has led to a decline in their use except in the augmentation of the alveolus in localised areas.

Calcium hydroxyapatite

The material in the form of granules 1mm in diameter is injected into a sub-mucoperiosteal pocket. This is developed through small vertical incisions in the canine region in the mandible or a single midline incision in the maxilla. A sub-periosteal pocket is developed by a process of tunnelling, into which the material can be injected. Initially the graft may be stabilised by ingrowth of fibrous tissue and new bone formation but migration of the material can reduce ridge height and obliterate the sulcus.

Implants

Advances in implant technology has seen predictable levels of success in replacement of dental units either to retain dentures in the edentulous or provide permanent replacements for lost units in the partly dentate patient. To achieve success careful patient selection, planning and preparation are essential. Patients should be healthy and well motivated, with adequate bone and healthy soft tissues, and should be capable of maintaining a high standard of oral hygiene as plaque and calculus will adhere to implants. A specialist in restorative dentistry should be involved in the planning and provision of the overlying superstructure. Many implant systems are available but those relying on osseointegration have the best success.

Osseointegration

This concept was first pioneered by Branemark in Sweden and is defined as a direct connection between living bone and a load-bearing endosseous implant when viewed at the light microscopic level. The main factors neccesary to achieve osseointegration are:

- A totally biocompatible implant material
- Precise adaptation of the implant to the bone
- An atraumatic surgical technique
- A period of unloaded healing

Biocompatible materials

The implant must not cause any form of foreign body reaction as this will lead to a weaker bone implant bond and possible rejection of the implant. Titanium implants have been shown to be bio-inert and are in common usage.

Precise adaptation

This is achieved using a series of implants matched to drill sizes to minimise the distance between the bone and the implant.

Atraumatic surgical technique

If any overheating of bone occurs during preparation of the implant site intra-bony alkaline phosphatasc is denatured with consequent reduction of alkaline calcium production. Bone overheating is controlled by the use of copious irrigation and low-speed high-torque drilling with sharp burs.

Unloaded healing

The provision of a close bone–implant interface relies on initial woven bone being replaced with lamellar bone. Any loading or movement of the implant in the early stages of healing may prevent this and lead to a fibrous interface. The first month following placement is most critical.

Surgery

The first stage of implant surgery is the placement of an implant under the mucoperiosteum flush with the alveolar crest. If insufficient bone is present to allow placement of an implant without perforating any vital structures such as the inferior dental canal, the nasal floor or the maxillary antrum bone grafting should be considered. The sinus lift procedure provides an increased depth of bone in the posterior maxilla.

The implant is covered by mucoperiosteum and left undisturbed for a period of 3–6 months while bone formation stabilises. The implant is then uncovered and the second stage of the implant is attached which then lies above the mucoperiosteum. The implant should be firm and stable and able to carry a superstructure onto which a prosthesis may be fitted.

Commonly four or five implants might be placed between the mental foramina to retain a prosthesis which is partly tissue borne. In the maxilla more

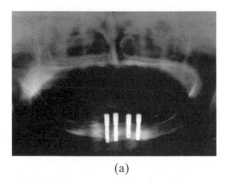
(a)

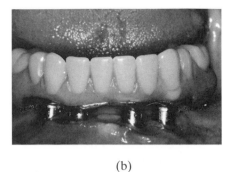
(b)

Fig. 11.7 Mandibular implants: (a) four titanium implants placed in an edentulous mandible – note they are positioned anterior to the mental nerve; (b) Prosthetic attachment in place on mandibular implants. Scrupulous oral hygiene must be maintained around the implant to reduce the chance of failure.

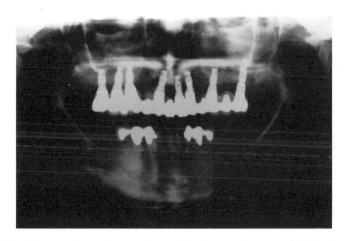

Fig. 11.8 Maxillary implants. Positioning of implants relies on available bone. Bone grafting may be necessary to place implants posteriorly.

posteriorly placed implants allow an improved design. Wherever they are placed a strict regime of oral hygiene must be maintained to minimise bone loss around the implant.

Further reading

Peterson, L.R., Ellis, E., Hupp, J.R. & Tucker, M.R. (1998) *Contemporary Oral and Maxillofacial Surgery*, 3rd edn. Mosby-Year Book, Missouri.

Chapter 12
Treatment of Surgical Infections in the Orofacial Region

- Acute infections
- Diagnosis
- Bacterial investigations
- Principles of treatment of acute infections
- Infections of the face, head and neck
- Chronic infections of the jaws

Acute infections

Acute infections of the orofacial region are due to the pathogenic activities of micro-organisms including viruses, fungi and bacteria. Surgical infection is mainly due to bacterial infection. The progress of any infection is governed by the host response to the invading organisms. Factors related to the organism that are important include their number and virulence. Organisms vary in their virulence and can be divided into:

- Commensals
- Potential pathogens
- Pathogens

Commensals

These may become pathogenic by a change of site or host resistance. Host factors that are important concerning the establishment of an infection include:

- Age (resistance is decreased at the extremes of age)
- Concurrent disease
- Drugs (immunosuppressants)
- Therapeutic irradiation (this decreases the local blood supply)

Spread of infection

Once established infection may spread and this is governed by host and pathogen factors. Local anatomy is an important host factor in the direction of

156

spread. There are three serious sequelae of spread of infection in the orofacial region:

- Airway obstruction
- Intracranial spread
- Septicaemia

Infection may spread by one of three routes:

- Tissue planes and spaces
- The lymphatics
- The blood

The prompt treatment of oral infection requires an understanding of both systemic and local factors.

Diagnosis

The diagnosis is made from the history and examination of the patient supported by additional special investigations. The five classical signs of acute infection are diagnostic:

- Swelling
- Redness
- Pain or tenderness
- Heat
- Loss of function

In addition, there may be a discharge of pus and regional lymphadenopathy. The systemic signs include:

- Raised temperature
- Rapid pulse
- General malaise

The typical picture of the acute phase may be altered where antibacterial drugs have been ineffectively used. They may not have overcome the infection but have produced a state of balance between the invading bacteria and the patient's defences.

The formation of pus in a superficial abscess causes softening with fluctuation, redness and marked tenderness at the centre of the inflamed area. In a deep abscess affecting the neck, pus may spread widely and fluctuance may be masked by tense, oedematous swelling in the overlying tissue, which can be indistinguishable from cellulitis. The patient's temperature continues to rise with a swinging temperature suggesting the presence of suppuration.

A clear and concise medical history is recorded with special regard to metabolic or blood disorders. In very acute, recurrent or persistent infections, special investigations should be performed such as:

- Urinalysis
- Haemoglobin
- Full blood count and differential white cell count–leucocytosis
- Fasting blood sugar
- Blood cultures
- Erythrocyte sedimentation rate

Radiographs may be uninformative in early acute infections of the jaw, unless there has been a previous chronic condition. Initially, a dental abscess may appear as a diffuse radiolucency associated with the apex of a non-vital tooth. After a period of approximately 10 days, bone changes may be seen as either localised periapical areas or more diffuse changes in the case of osteomyelitis.

The underlying cause such as a non-vital tooth should be sought although treatment should not be delayed until the cause is found.

From the history the clinician should record:

- Duration of infection
- Changes in signs and symptoms
- Sequence of events
- Treatments sought including antibiotics prescribed

From the examination the clinician should record:

- Swelling, diffuse or localised (fluctuant)
- Lymphadenopathy
- Trismus
- Presence of sinus
- Changes in the jaws and teeth
- Presence of pyrexia (body temperature)

Bacterial investigations

Microbiological investigation can play an important role in the management of a patient with orofacial suppurative infection. All efforts should be made to obtain an appropriate specimen for any patient suspected of having a bacterial infection. Within the laboratory the organisms will be cultured, identified and an indication given of the drugs to which the bacteria will be sensitive.

Culture and sensitivity

This is imperative where there is:

- Rapidly spreading infection
- Infection in the medically compromised patient
- Infection not responding to antibiotic therapy
- Recurrent infection

- Osteomyelitis
- Post-operative infection

Methods of sampling

Aspiration

Where collections of pus have not discharged, aspiration is preferred to prevent loss of oxygen-sensitive strict anaerobes prior to processing. The overlying tissue is first thoroughly cleaned and dried. An 18 gauge needle in a syringe is inserted into the most dependent part of the swelling and a sample aspirated. The sample should be immediately sealed to avoid drying and contamination from the air and sent to the laboratory accompanied by the appropriate microbiology form with the date and time of collection, nature and site of the sample, method of collection, current and previous antibiotic therapy, together with any relevant clinical information. Culture and sensitivity results should be available within 36 to 48 hours.

Swabs

A bacteriological swab may be used for taking pus either from an extra-oral sinus or from an abscess drained through an extra-oral incision providing that the skin and surrounding area have been thorough cleansed beforehand. However, swabs taken inside the mouth are liable to contamination from the saliva so that growths obtained are often reported as mixed oral flora. Swabbing is the least reliable method for obtaining a specimen for culture and sensitivity, but may be required when aspiration is unsuccessful.

Principles of treatment of acute infections

The management of an infection relies on general and local measures.

General measures

The general care of patients has been discussed in Chapter 2.

Rest

Where there is an elevated temperature, the patient should rest in bed. When there is gross swelling of the neck or floor of the mouth, or the patient is toxic, he should be admitted to hospital.

Nutritional support

Copious fluids are administered to combat dehydration, which is a complication of high fever. Circulating toxins are diluted and their excretion encouraged by an increased turnover of water.

Diet

A balanced diet of easily digested proteins and carbohydrates is required (Chapter 2).

Analgesia

Orofacial infections are painful and an important part of management is good pain control. Non-steroidal analgesics are the drugs of choice, many of which have the benefit of being anti-pyretic. In the case of airway problems any drugs with a respiratory depressant effect such as opioids should be avoided.

Control of infection

Antibacterial drugs are not always necessary in the treatment of infections. Drainage, removal of the cause, and applications of heat may be enough to enable the patient to overcome the condition and antibiotics must not be prescribed to replace or delay these local measures.

Indications for antibiotic therapy

- Where culture and sensitivity has been obtained
- Continuing unresponsive infection
- Systemic spread
- Chronic infections
- Post-surgical infections in medically compromised or debilitated patients
- Post-operative infections at the operative site

Unfortunately in many of these situations it is not feasible to await the result of a culture and thus antibiotics are often prescribed blind. Amoxycillin, which is a broad spectrum penicillin, is often the preferred drug. A loading dose of 3 g amoxycillin orally rapidly achieves bactericidal concentrations in the blood, and may be followed by 250 mg or 500 mg eight hourly. Metronidazole (200–400 mg eight hourly) targets anaerobic bacteria which are often the causative organisms in many dental infections. A combination of amoxycillin with metronidazole may be appropriate in more severe infections and it may be necessary to admit the patient to provide antimicrobial therapy intravenously, together with surgical drainage. Once an antibiotic has been prescribed it should not be changed within the first 48 hours unless there is bacteriological evidence of resistance. If clinical improvement is occurring despite laboratory evidence of resistance it is not essential to change the regimen. There is no set duration of administration of antibiotics and no rationale in 'completing the course'. Antibiotic therapy should not be maintained after clinical resolution has occurred. Hyperbaric oxygen therapy is useful in promoting bone healing. It increases the effectiveness of antibiotics and the vascularity of tissues which have been subjected to radiation therapy.

Local measures

Local measures include:

- Removal of the cause
- Institution of drainage
- Prevention of spread
- Restoration of function

Removal of the cause

This is the most important principle in the management of infection. In well-localised minor infections it may immediately cure the condition. In other cases it may initially be simpler to institute drainage and prevent spread. However, if the cause is not removed infection will recur. Causes of orofacial bacterial infections include:

- Necrotic pulps
- Periodontal disease
- Avascular bony remnants (sequestrae)
- Foreign bodies
- Salivary calculi

Institution of drainage

Reddening of the skin, fluctuation and a point of maximum tenderness indicate localisation of pus (pointing). When this occurs the pus must be drained and a surgical incision leaves much less scarring than if pus bursts through the skin spontaneously. To be effective, drainage must be provided at the lowest point of the abscess. A drain (Fig. 7.6) should always be inserted to keep the opening patent for as long as the discharge continues. In cellulitis drainage is not established until the condition has localised, usually after 3 or 4 days. However, where a brawny, spreading swelling of the floor of the mouth and neck might involve the larynx and jeopardise the airway, surgery will reduce the tension in the tissue spaces and should not be withheld.

Intraoral incisions

In the mucous membrane incisions are made parallel to the occlusal surface of the teeth, 1 to 2 cm in length, with due regard for underlying structures such as the mental nerve. Smaller incisions are ineffective.

Extraoral incisions

Incisions through skin should avoid the branches of the facial nerve. Where the abscess is deep and a free discharge is not obtained through a simple skin incision, Hilton's method of blunt dissection is performed. This involves inserting closed sinus forceps into the wound, which are then opened slowly but firmly to separate the soft tissue planes; the forceps are then withdrawn open to avoid damaging nerves or vessels by closing them blind. This procedure is repeated until the abscess is reached and pus discharges. In dental infections an area of rough cortical bone can be felt on the mandible or maxilla where the periosteum has been raised.

Prevention of spread

This is achieved by rest, drainage and the use of antimicrobial drugs. Rest of the affected part may be difficult when dealing with the oro-facial region. However trismus, when present, achieves this naturally.

Restoration of function

The patient should be reviewed following the acute phase to ensure that function is restored. Trismus may persist and require treatment to improve mouth opening (Chapter 17) and dental units may require restoration or replacement. Other causes such as periodontal disease or sialadenitis should be treated to prevent recurrence.

Timing

The decision when to perform various procedures is of great importance and requires considerable experience. In acute infection with a high temperature, immediate treatment with antibacterial drugs should be commenced. If pus has localised this must be drained without delay and culture and sensitivity tests performed. Antibacterial drugs can be started blind and continued until the results of the sensitivity tests are available. If not possible before, the cause should be removed as soon as the acute phase has passed.

Maintenance of the airway

Infections in the neck may cause oedema of the glottis with acute respiratory embarrassment. In all acute swellings where swallowing is difficult patients should be watched for signs of difficulty in breathing and everything necessary for emergency tracheotomy should be at hand. To maintain control of the airway an awake bronchoscopic intubation may be neccesary as a general anaesthetic may precipitate respiratory arrest when the accessory muscles of respiration stop functioning. Anaesthesia may be induced after control of the airway has been achieved.

Common infections in the mouth

Pericoronitis

Pericoronitis presents as inflammation around the crown of an erupting or partly erupted, but impacted, tooth. In adults it is common in the mandible,

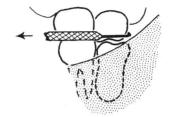

Fig. 12.1 As it is often difficult to see if the upper third molar is biting on the inflamed gingival flap over a partly erupted lower third molar, a dental probe may be placed distal to the upper third molar and drawn forward over its occlusal surface with the teeth in occlusion. This will not be possible where the upper cusps are in contact with the swollen gum flap.

particularly associated with the lower third molar tooth. The causes of the inflammation are:

- Infection
- Trauma from an opposing tooth
- Foreign body reaction due to food packing

An acute attack may be precipitated by the upper third molar traumatising the operculum of the lower third molar (Fig. 12.1), which then becomes infected. The patient complains of pain and tenderness in the operculum and a foul taste. When severe there is swelling of the floor of mouth and face, with trismus. There may be difficulty in swallowing and a raised temperature. The condition is rare in the maxilla.

Diagnosis

Diagnosis is made after confirming the presence of the impacted tooth with radiographs, and eliminating apical or periodontal disease in neighbouring teeth.

Treatment

Treatment is in two stages, directed first to the infection and second to the impacted tooth. For the acute inflammation hourly hot salt water mouth baths held over the affected operculum should be carried out. It is essential to eliminate any trauma from the opposing tooth. Where the upper tooth is non-functional it can be extracted at once under local anaesthesia, providing access is satisfactory, but where the tooth is functional the cusps may be ground clear of the operculum. If the temperature is raised or trismus is present, antibacterial drugs are prescribed. Spread of the infection from this site can quickly involve tissue spaces close to the airway (Fig. 12.2), and prompt and effective treatment is essential. The surgical treatment of the impacted tooth may have to be delayed until the acute phase, particularly the trismus, has resolved, which may take some 2–3 weeks, but consideration should be given to immediate removal of the tooth as this will institute drainage and remove the cause.

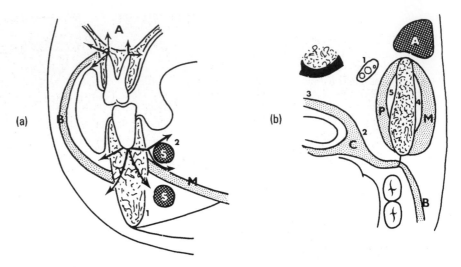

Fig. 12.2   Spread of infection: (a) Coronal section through the tissue spaces of the face and neck. Note *A* the maxillary sinus, *B* the buccinator muscle, *M* the mylohyoid muscle, *S* the submandibular salivary gland. Spaces shown are (1) the submandibular and (2) the sublingual. (b) Transverse section through the tissue spaces of the face and neck. Note *A* the parotid salivary gland, *B* the buccinator muscle, *C* the superior constrictor muscle, *M* the masseter muscle, *P* the medial pterygoid muscle and (1) the carotid sheath. Spaces shown are (2) the lateral pharyngeal, (3) the retro-pharyngeal, (4) the submasseteric, (5) the pterygomandibular.

Operculectomy has been practised but the results are unsatisfactory and it is to be condemned except where the tooth will erupt into a functional occlusion.

Acute periapical abscess without soft tissue involvement

Periapical infection from non-vital teeth or periodontal disease may either be contained and present as a low-grade chronic condition or apical granuloma with mild symptoms, or may suppurate to form an acute periapical abscess.

Diagnosis

The patient with an acute periapical abscess will complain of severe pain and the affected tooth feels raised in its socket. At first the pain may be eased by biting on the tooth but later it becomes exquisitely tender to touch. Examination at an early stage shows no involvement of the oral mucosa or soft tissue and systemic symptoms are usually absent.

Treatment

Where it is hoped to retain the tooth, the root canal is opened through the crown to provide drainage and access for root canal therapy. Otherwise the tooth may be extracted.

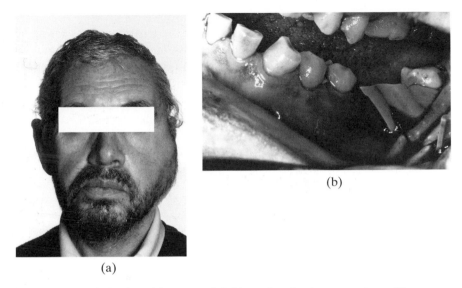

(b)

(a)

Fig. 12.3 Acute infection: (a) acute painful buccal and submasseteric swelling associated with grossly carious lower molar; (b) intraoral drainage following tooth removal.

Subperiosteal abscess and spread into the soft tissues

Pus from an acute periapical abscess takes the track of least resistance through the medullary bone and points on the nearest epithelial surface. This is usually the buccal aspect of the maxilla or mandible where the alveolar bone is thinnest. Pus breaks through the bone above or below the attachment of buccinator. This determines whether the discharge occurs intraorally or through the soft tissues onto the skin of the face (Fig. 12.2).

In the maxilla the lateral incisor and palatal roots of the molar teeth commonly present as palatal abscesses. Anterior teeth may discharge into the nose and posterior teeth into the maxillary sinus. In the mandible the relationship of the roots to the insertion of mylohyoid determines where lingual discharge will occur. The apices of the lower third molar and on occasions the second molar lie below the insertion of mylohyoid and thus pointing on the skin can occur. The remaining apices lying above mylohyoid cause discharge into the floor of the mouth. Periapical abscesses can discharge through the root canal or periodontal membrane.

Presentation and diagnosis

The cardinal signs of acute inflammation with mild systemic symptoms are present. Initially there is a tense very painful subperiosteal swelling near to the tooth with some facial oedema. Pain reduction usually occurs once pus is released through the mucoperiosteum into the mouth or through the periosteum into the soft tissues of the face and neck.

Treatment

If there is inflammatory oedema present the treatment is as for an acute peri-apical abscess. Pus below the mucoperiosteum is unlikely to drain through an extraction socket and must be incised and drained. Systemic symptoms necessitate the need for antibiotic therapy (Fig. 12.3).

Infections of the face, head and neck

Spread of infection via tissue spaces, the lymphatics and blood may lead to the serious consequences of airway obstruction, intracranial spread and septicaemia.

Spread through muscle and fascial planes

Spread of infection takes place through potential spaces, normally filled with loose areolar tissue. These spaces lie between muscles, bones and viscera that are covered by condensations of fascia which form strong fibrous sheaths. The fascial planes of importance are:

- Deep cervical
- Pre-tracheal
- Pre-vertebral
- Carotid sheath

Deep cervical fascia

The superficial layer encloses the neck and prevents deep infections pointing easily onto the skin. Arising from the scapula, clavicle and manubrium sterni it sweeps up the neck as a continuous tube attached, posteriorly to the ligamentum nuchae, anteriorly to the hyoid bone. It divides at the lower border of the mandible to form the submandibular space and is then attached lingually to the mylohyoid line and buccally to the outer aspect of the mandible. Buccally the fascia is then reflected up onto the zygomatic arch where posteriorly it ensheaths the parotid gland and is inserted into the mastoid process and the superior nuchal line on the skull. Invaginations are formed in the neck; the pre-tracheal fascia, a continuation of the deep surface, which invests the trachea and thyroid gland; the prevertebral fascia, lying anterior to the prevertebral muscles; and the carotid sheath, which surrounds the great vessels of the neck. All these extend down into the thorax and can provide a pathway for spread of infection to the mediastinum. A number of potential tissue spaces exist in the neck and orofacial region through which infection may spread:

- Sublingual space
- Submental space
- Submandibular space
- Pterygomandibular space
- Lateral pharyngeal space

- Retropharyngeal space
- Infratemporal space
- Submasseteric space

Sublingual space

Two spaces on the medial aspect of the mandible lying above mylohyoid, both continuous across the midline and bounded by the insertion of the suprahyoid muscles into the hyoid bone. A superficial space lying between mylohyoid and geniohyoid, and a deep space between geniohyoid and genioglossus. Infection can track laterally across the floor of the mouth or posteriorly to cause inflammatory oedema of the larynx and respiratory embarrassment. The deep part of the submandibular gland lies in the sublingual space and curves round and down below the mylohyoid muscle to allow communication between the sublingual and submandibular spaces (Fig. 12.2a).

Submental space

Submental space below the chin drains to the submandibular spaces.

Submandibular spaces

These are continuous across the midline and are bounded by the deep cervical fascia laterally and the mylohyoid muscle superiorly. The superficial part of the submandibular gland lies in this space. Infection can track from the lower molars and contralateral space, which communicates with the fascial planes of the pharynx and neck (Fig. 12.4).

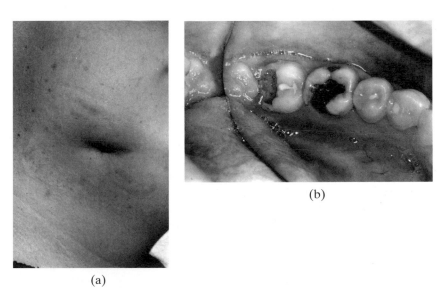

(b)

(a)

Fig. 12.4 Chronic infection: (a) extraoral submandibular sinus associated with; (b) grossly carious lower molar.

Pterygomandibular space

This lies between the medial aspect of the ascending ramus and the medial ptery-goid muscle and is limited superiorly by the lateral pterygoid muscle. It communicates with the lateral pharyngeal and infratemporal spaces (Fig. 12.2b).

Lateral pharygeal space

The boundaries of this space are: medially the superior pharyngeal constrictor muscle, laterally the medial pterygoid muscle and anteriorly the pterygo-mandibular raphe where the fascia covering superior constrictor is reflected onto the medial pterygoid muscle.

Posteriorly lies the styloid process and stylohyoid and stylopharyngeous muscles, along which infection can spread to the larynx. It is close to the carotid sheath and communicates with the submandibular and sublingual spaces round the submandibular salivary gland, the posterior part of which protrudes into the lateral pharyngeal space. The submandibular gland can play an important part in the spread of infection as it links the submandibular, sublingual and lateral pharyngeal spaces (Fig. 12.2).

Retropharyngeal space

Lying between the constrictor muscles of the pharynx and prevertcbral muscles this connects the right and left lateral pharyngeal spaces (Fig. 12.2b).

Infratemporal space

This is bounded anteriorly by the maxillary tuberosity, medially by the lateral pterygoid plate and inferior belly of the lateral pterygoid muscle and laterally by the tendon of temporalis and the coronoid process.

Submasseteric space

This is a potential space between masseter and the lateral aspect of the mandible.

Lymphatic drainage

Scalp and facial skin drains into the superficial group of nodes in a circle around the head. These are the occipital, posterior auricular, parotid, and facial nodes. Efferent vessels from these pass down to the superior lymph glands of the deep cervical chain. Submental lymph nodes lie between the anterior bellies of the two digastric muscles and drain the lower lip and incisor region of the mandible. Anterior tongue and floor of mouth lymph then passes to the submandibular nodes or direct to the deep cervical chain. Submandibular lymph nodes lie in the submandibular triangle and drain the remaining ipsilateral lymph vessels of the lips, cheeks, tongue and jaws, and thence to the deep cervical nodes accompanying the internal jugular vein. The anterior mouth drains to the lower group of nodes in this chain whilst the posterior mouth drains to the upper group of nodes. Pathological conditions of the tonsil and mouth may result in early enlargement of the jugulodigastric node (superior nodes) at the level of the posterior belly of the digastric.

The response of the lymphatic system varies with the severity of the infection. Acute infections lead to lymphangitis – inflammation. Organisms and their toxins in the node lead to lymphadenitis (enlargement). Virulent infections may lead to suppuration and abcess formation in the node. It is important to exclude other possible causes of lymph node enlargement.

Spread via the bloodstream

Entry of infected material into the bloodstream can lead to septicaemia or toxaemia. These are potentially life-threatening conditions. In addition the intravenous route is a means of intracranial entry.

Intracranial spread of infection

From an intraoral source this may lead to:

- Cavernous sinus thrombosis
- Brain abscess

Cavernous sinus thrombosis

Although rare, this is a serious condition. The sinus may be infected by general spread in the blood either via the angular veins of the orbit (following infection from a maxillary anterior tooth) or by a short venous connection from the pterygoid plexus (from posterior maxillary teeth). Among the structures which pass through this sinus are the nerves which supply the muscles of the orbit, branches of the trigeminal nerve and the internal carotid artery. The presenting eye signs are:

- Opthalmoplegia (inability to move the eye)
- Ptosis (drooping upper eye-lid)
- Proptosis (extrusion of the eye)

Brain abscess

Direct entry of infected material may occur via tissue planes, access to the brain being achieved along the carotid sheath. Another route is via the nasal sinuses following infection of an upper molar tooth gaining access to the maxillary sinus. Once here, spread to other nasal sinuses may occur and breach of a sinus wall in contact with the brain can result in intra-cranial spread.

Maxillary infections

Where pus points buccally above the buccinator it will form an abscess in the cheek and may spread over a wide area as there is nothing to contain it. Those from the anterior teeth cause an infraorbital abscess which is serious because thrombosis of the facial vein may follow. This vessel anastomoses with orbital veins which drain into the cavernous sinus. In this way infection may pass from the face into the cavernous sinus.

Abscesses in the cheek may point anywhere on the face, and when drained the incision is made parallel to the branches of the facial nerve. Infection of the infratemporal space may be caused by posterior superior dental nerve injections given behind the tuberosity of the maxilla or by spread from the maxillary third molar tooth. This space may be drained intraorally through the buccal sulcus lateral and posterior to the tuberosity.

Mandibular infections

Spread of infection buccally, below the attachment of the buccinator, causes a swelling in the cheek over the lateral aspect of the mandible, but the inferior border of the bone remains palpable if the submandibular space is not involved. Incision for drainage may have to be made over the lateral aspect of the mandible.

An infection in the submandibular space gives rise to swelling over the lower border of the mandible and into the neck. It is drained by an incision parallel with the lower border of the mandible and about 2 cm below it to avoid the mandibular branch of the facial nerve and the facial vessels.

The sublingual spaces are involved when spread takes place above the mylohyoid into the floor of the mouth, which becomes swollen and is raised with difficulty in swallowing. These spaces may be drained by an incision in the floor of the mouth but, if the submandibular space is also involved, an extraoral approach is more satisfactory.

Infection of the pterygomandibular space, with symptoms of trismus and pain on swallowing, may follow an inferior dental nerve injection or spread of infection from the lower third molar tooth. This space and the submandibular space communicate with the lateral pharyngeal space which, if involved, gives rise to swelling in the lateral wall of the oro-pharynx, and mesial and posterior to the angle of the mandible, accompanied by trismus and difficulty in swallowing.

The lateral pharyngeal, and through it the pterygomandibular space, may be drained by an incision made 2 cm below the angle of the mandible. In those rare cases where only the pterygomandibular space is affected it may be opened by incising down the anterior border of the ascending ramus intraorally.

Infection from the lower third molar tooth may also occasionally track buccally either under the skin superficial to the masseter or less often into the submassetric space (Fig. 12.2b).

Ludwig's angina

This presents as bilateral submandibular and sublingual cellulitis. The swelling is board hard and the tongue is lifted upwards and forwards by the swelling and may protrude through the teeth. Trismus may be severe. Infection may spread to the lateral pharyngeal spaces and down to the larynx, to cause oedema of the glottis and asphyxia, or to the thorax via the carotid sheath or to the cavernous sinus via the pterygoid venous plexus. Severe cases may require tracheotomy.

The cellulitis is treated by intravenous antibiotics and bilateral 'through and through' drains from external incisions into the floor of the mouth. The incisions are made below the lower molar regions of the jaw and blunt dissection using Hilton's method is performed up to second incisions in the floor of the mouth. The drains are brought from intra- to extraoral. Pus is seldom found but the congestion is usually relieved.

Osteomyelitis

Osteomyelitis is an infection involving all layers of bone in which widespread necrosis may occur. It is rare in the maxilla due to the rich blood supply but on occasions may affect the anterior palate where the bone is thicker. It is more common in the mandible, usually as a result of dental infection, trauma or a blood-borne infection. Development depends on highly virulent organisms, low patient resistance and lack of drainage. The incidence has been reduced by antibiotic therapy. The presentation of chronic inflammatory swellings complicated by subacute episodes is more common, which may be settled by a long period of antibiotic therapy. Short courses of antibiotics may suppress but not cure, contributing to extensive destruction of bone.

Presentation

Pus tracks through the medulla of bone (rather than through a narrow track into the soft tissue). It reaches the cortical plate at several points to lift the periosteum and deprive large areas of the blood supply. Pus may then discharge through a sinus and the situation enters a chronic phase. Limitation of the infection is achieved by osteoclasts separating away the dead bone (sequestrum) which is walled off by granulation tissue. Osteoblasts initiate repair and support of the weakened bone by laying down a new layer of bone – (involucrum). Discharge continues until the sequestrum is removed. If drainage is inadequate, slow spread with formation of new sequestra may continue indefinitely.

Diagnosis

Symptoms can include those of acute infection, severe pain, pyrexia, teeth tender to percussion and loose, intermittent mental sensory loss in the mandible. Facial swelling soon follows, followed by discharge of pus and sinus formation. Bare rough bone is palpable at base of sinus.

Radiographs are initially negative but after 10 days irregular radiolucent areas are seen. Later, sequestra appear as radiopacities surrounded by a radiolucent zone. Bone destruction may lead to pathological fracture visible on radiographs.

Treatment

Immediate admission to hospital is advisable. High dose antibiotics and the establishment of drainage via an extraoral incision are the priorities. Only very loose or non-vital teeth should be removed whilst the application of heat should be avoided as it may lead to spread of infection. Hyperbaric oxygen may be useful and antibiotics are continued for at least 14 days after disease has settled.

Sequestrectomy

Removal of sequestra under antibiotic cover is an essential part of treatment. A clear radiolucent line around the sequestra on radiograph should suggest simple removal of the sequestrum. Sequestra above the inferior alveolar canal may be removed intra-orally with the resultant defect packed open. Lower border sequestra require a lower border incision; where a sinus is present incorporate this in the incision line. Non-vital bone is excised and the area gently curetted to expose healthy bleeding bone; a drain is placed.

Mowlem's decorticectomy involves removal of the thick poorly vascularised buccal plate over the diseased area, which promotes ingrowth of granulation tissue and speeds wound healing.

Acute necrotising fasciitis

This rapidly spreading and aggressive infection of fascia and muscles presents following trauma or post-surgery in debilitated patients. The skin is mottled and dusky with sloughing. Both aerobic and anaerobic organisms are involved and management consists of drainage, debridement of necrotic tissue and high dose intravenous antibiotics.

Mediastinitis

This very severe infection may spread through orofacial fascial spaces via the deep cervical spaces to affect the mediastinum. This presents as fever, chest pain, general malaise and a raised temperature. Management is tailored to remove the source. Incision and drainage of cervical spaces and mediastinal drainage with long term high doses of antibiotics are necessary. There is a high level of morbidity and mortality with the possible sequelae of damage to large vessels and cardiac failure.

Acute maxillary infection in children

A rare, acute staphylococcal infection affects the maxilla, usually in infants a few weeks old.

Aetiology

The infection follows birth trauma, mouth abrasions or blood-borne infection.

Presentation and diagnosis

The disease is of rapid onset with all the signs of acute infection. The child is very ill with a high temperature, swelling of the cheek with eye closure, pus discharge from the nostrils and/or intraoral sinuses. Partially calcified teeth may be devitalised and sequestrate. Occasionally thicker bony margins, such as the infraorbital margin may sequestrate. Radiographs are not helpful as the maxilla, at this age, consists of thin bone around a 'bag of teeth'.

Treatment

The patient should be admitted under the care of a paediatrician for antibiotics and drainage. Later any sequestra (bone, teeth) may require removal to avoid a chronic phase.

Osteomyelitis in children

This may occur acutely in the mandible following exanthematous fevers, tonsillitis, sinusitis or middle ear disease. Symptoms are similar to those of the adult. Unerupted teeth may be exfoliated and complications include involvement of growth centres and subsequent deformity or ankylosis of the joint. Treatment is as for an adult.

Chronic infections of the jaws

Chronic periapical abscess

An acute periapical abscess can become chronic if the cause is not removed and it drains through a sinus. Sinus blockage may contribute to acute exacerbations. Treatment includes extraction or root canal therapy with or without subsequent apicectomy. On rare occasions extraoral sinuses may occur which if unsightly may require excision (Fig. 12.4).

Tuberculosis

Tuberculosis is now more common, particularly in immigrant populations. It may spread to the mouth in infected sputum or by the haematogenous route, usually secondary to lung infection. The causal organism is mycobacterium tuberculosis. Cervical tuberculous adenitis may be a primary infection, presenting as enlarged non-tender lymph nodes.

Presentation and diagnosis

The tongue is often affected with deep ragged painful ulcers. Smears from mouth ulcers should be cultured and the chest radiographed for other foci of infection. Osteomyelitis of the jaw can occur, characterised by long-standing localised tender swellings which may discharge at the lower border of the mandible. Sequestra may be present and secondary infection may occur.

Treatment

This is first directed to the general care of the patient. Local measures include antibiotics, drainage and sequestrectomy where appropriate. Drugs such as isoniazid, rifampicin and pyrazinamide are administered and routine sputum and wound cultures are carried out.

Actinomycosis

This is a chronic infection caused by *Actinomyces israelii* which may affect the face and neck, the lungs or abdomen.

Diagnosis

The patient complains of a 'board' hard, lumpy swelling usually over the angle of the mandible. It is sometimes bluish in colour and tends to form multiple sinuses which discharge pus containing 'sulphur granules'. These, if examined microscopically, show the organisms.

Sometimes the disease occurs as a mixed infection and presents as a typical acute abscess which fails to clear up normally. In these cases frequent anaerobic cultures should be made as there is often difficulty in isolating the organisms and the diagnosis cannot be definitely established without a positive culture. Rarely is the bone also involved.

Treatment

Antibacterial drugs are prescribed, for a period of 4–6 weeks. Surgery is limited to draining superficial lesions, but if bone is involved the affected area may be curetted and packed open and the teeth involved extracted.

Further reading

Ingham, H.R., Kalbag, R.M., Tharagonnet, D., High, A.S., Sengupta, R.P. & Selkon, J.B. (1978) Abscesses of the frontal lobe of the brain secondary to convert dental sepsis. *Lancet*, **2**, 8088.

Iwu, G.O. (1990) Ludwig's angina: report of seven cases and review of current concepts on management. *British Journal Oral and Maxillofacial Surgery*, **28**, 189.

Lewis, M.A.O., MacFarlane, T.W. & McGowan, D.A. (1990) A microbiological and clinical review of the acute dentoalveolar abscess. *British Journal Oral Maxillofacial Surg*ery, **28**, 359.

Rud, J. (1970) Removal of impacted lower third molars with acute pericoronitis and necrotising gingivitis. *Br. J. Oral Surg.*, **7**(3), 153–60.

Chapter 13
Treatment of Cysts of the Jaw

- Diagnosis
- Treatment
- Developmental cysts of non-dental origin
- Non-epithelial lined cysts
- Soft-tissue cysts

A cyst may be defined as a radiolucency which is usually fluid filled and has a lining. The lining is frequently epithelium and in the mouth is either of dental or non-dental origin. A cyst must be differentiated from other pathology that might mimic it, particularly neoplasia.

The common cysts of the jaw arising from epithelium of dental origin are:

- Dental or periodontal cysts
- Residual cysts
- Dentigerous cysts
- Eruption cysts
- Keratocysts

Dental or periodontal cysts

These form from the epithelial cells or rests of Malassez which are the remnants of Hertwig's sheath. They remain throughout life, scattered in clusters, in the periodontal membrane. Chronic infection may stimulate them to proliferate and form epithelial lined cysts in the jaws. These occur chiefly over the apex of a dead tooth, but may occasionally be found on its lateral aspect, when they are called lateral periodontal cysts.

Residual cysts

These occur in edentulous areas of the jaws and are dental cysts believed to have been present before the dead tooth was extracted and which continue to grow.

Dentigerous cysts

These form between the reduced enamel epithelium of the follicle around a developing tooth and its crown.

Eruption cysts

These are cysts forming over erupting teeth. Those over deciduous or permanent teeth with no deciduous predecessor are believed to originate from the cells of the enamel organ. Where there has been a deciduous predecessor the epithelial rests of Malassez from this tooth could give rise to one of these cysts.

The above cysts of dental origin are believed to increase in size either from continual liquefaction of their shed cells (which forms the cholesterol that gives the contents a characteristic golden appearance) or as a result of the positive osmotic pressure of the hypertonic contents which draws water in from the tissues.

Keratocysts (primordial cysts)

These are said to arise from the dental lamina or from the enamel organ of a tooth germ. Their lining is of well-differentiated epithelium which may show ortho- or para-keratosis. They are believed to increase in size by mural division. Beneath the epithelium is thin fibrous tissue which is easily torn and satellite cysts lying outside the main body of the lesion are often found. For these reasons keratocysts are well known to be difficult to eradicate and likely to recur after treatment. The recurrence rate has been reported to be 20–60%. The complete removal of all the lining of these cysts to avoid recurrence is of great importance. Their contents have less soluble protein (below 5 g per 100 ml) than dental cysts.

Diagnosis

Diagnosis can be difficult as, in many cases, the presentation is on routine radiograph. Histological confirmation of any diagnosis should be vigorously pursued.

History

The patient often gives no history as many cysts may escape attention until they become infected. Larger cysts may cause swelling of the jaw or face which in the edentulous may be associated with difficulty in wearing dentures. In the mandible, pressure on the inferior dental nerve almost never gives rise to mental anesthesia or paraesthesia, an important point in differentiation from tumours. Occasionally cysts reach such proportions that excessive resorption of bone leads to pathological fracture. Eventually the majority of cysts become infected with acute symptoms and, in those which have expanded into the soft tissues, an increase in the swelling.

Examination

An eruption cyst presents as a small blue swelling in the gum over an unerupted tooth. Uninfected dental, residual, or dentigerous cysts are painless and non-tender on palpation. When they are small and enclosed in bone they show no change in the form of the alveolus. Larger cysts cause a marked, smooth, rounded expansion of the bone, which may be reduced to a thin layer of corti-cal plate. This, if pressed, is resilient and may give rise to egg-shell crackling. In the mandible this expansion is said to take place buccally only, but occasionally it is seen lingually as well. Where the cyst has invaded the soft tissues the swelling is found to be fluctuant and a definite thrill can be made to pass through it. At this stage, if the mucous membrane covering is thin, it will have a bluish colour. Infected cysts have all the classical signs of acute infection and may present with a sinus discharging pus.

Missing teeth must be charted and the standing teeth carefully examined for caries, periodontal disease and mobility. A dentigerous cyst may be suspected where a tooth is missing from the arch without any history of previous extrac-tion. Dead and root-filled teeth are associated with dental cysts. The vitality of all teeth near the lesion must be tested with an electric pulp tester and the results compared with similar teeth on the unaffected side. If there is any delay between diagnosis and operation these tests should be repeated immediately before operation, for cysts not only arise from dead teeth but their expansion may also devitalise adjacent teeth.

Keratocysts may present like dental cysts but occur most commonly in the lower third molar region or distal to it and invade the ascending ramus exten-sively. They tend to expand anteroposteriorly in the medullary bone of the mandible and reach some size with minimal expansion of the cortical plate. Diagnosis may result from an infective episode or as a result of discovery on a scanning radiograph (Fig. 13.1). Multiple recurrent keratocysts are associated with basal cell carcinomas and some skeletal abnormalities in Gorlin–Goltz syn-drome. These patients require careful management and appropriate referral when necessary.

Radiography

Intraoral apical films usually suffice for small cysts. Larger ones may need extraoral and occlusal views of the jaws to show their full extent. This is demon-strated by radiographs taken in two planes, as treatment planning depends on a clear understanding of their size and their relationship to those vital struc-tures on which they may encroach.

Cysts appear as rounded, radiolucent areas sharply demarcated from normal bone by a thin, radiopaque, limiting line of compact bone (Fig. 13.1). This line is not usually present on radiographs of apical granulomas and is often absent or hazy round infected cysts. Apical periodontal cysts are associated with the

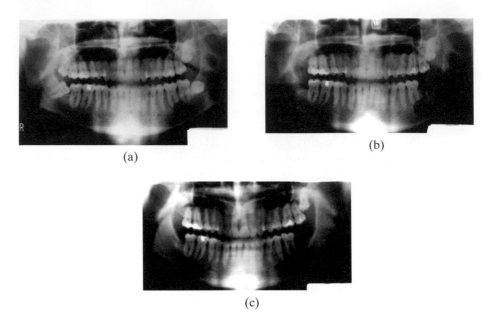

(a)

(b)

(c)

Fig. 13.1 Keratocyst: (a) at presentation; note resorption of apex of first molar; (b) Immediate postoperative appearance; (c) Appearance at six months showing bone healing. Inferior alveolar nerve function was not affected.

roots of dead teeth and may throw a shadow over, or displace, the roots of neighbouring teeth which, though apparently involved, may yet still be vital. Dental cysts, particularly the keratocyst, if loculated may simulate ameloblastoma or central giant cell reparative granuloma.

In the maxilla it is sometimes difficult to tell whether a radiolucent area is a cyst or a locule of the maxillary sinus. Therefore it is necessary to compare the radiographs with those of the opposite side; if a similar locule is present the radiolucent area is probably part of the sinus. If all the teeth are standing and vital, a cyst is unlikely to be present. Finally, where doubts still exist, the area may be aspirated and if air, not fluid, is withdrawn it is certainly part of the maxillary sinus.

Radiopaque fluids

Where the size and relations of a cyst are in doubt its contents may be aspirated and radiopaque fluid introduced. In large cavities it may only be possible to replace a proportion of the cyst contents, but the boundaries can be defined by taking radiographs with the head tilted in different positions so that the radiopaque medium lies against the doubtful margins.

Aspiration

An aspirating syringe with a broad bore needle is used, as the contents can be quite thick. Uninfected cysts should not be aspirated more than 24 hours before operation to avoid introducing infection. In those covered by thick bone it may be better delayed till, at operation, a flap has been laid back and bone removed.

All cysts of any size should be aspirated before operation. It is an important diagnostic measure which can save the surgeon much embarrassment from accidentally opening a solid tumour, or worse a central haemangioma. Microscopic examination of the aspirate may show the presence of cholesterol.

Further, only in this way may a keratocyst be differentiated from other odontogenic cysts before operation. This is done by electrophoresis of the aspirate which for keratocysts will show less than 5 g in 100 ml of soluble protein whereas other dental cysts will have quantities similar to that in the patient's serum.

Differential diagnosis

These lesions may all mimic cysts in their radiographic appearance:

- Solitary bone cyst
- Stafne's bone cavity
- Aneurysmal bone cyst
- Central giant cell granuloma
- Ameloblastoma
- Myeloma

Where doubt exists, blood chemistry, aspiration and biopsy should be performed.

Assessment

This includes an estimation of their size and, particularly in the mandible, the extent of bone resorption. Should there be a risk of a pathological fracture, the means to reduce and internally fix the mandible should be available (see Chapter 14). Many cysts, however, which on lateral radiographs occupy the whole of the depth of the mandible, usually have a sturdy lingual plate which adequately maintains the continuity of the bone through the operation.

The relationship of the cyst to adjacent structures is more important. Vital teeth which have a satisfactory periodontal condition and are functional, should be preserved. Consideration should be given to retaining dead teeth in well-cared-for mouths. This may be done by root-filling and apicectomy providing that at the very least the whole of the coronal half of the root is firmly held in sound alveolar bone. Dead teeth should be extracted where they are non-functional, mobile, the periodontal condition is poor and the patient already wears denture. Where a diagnosis of keratocyst has been confirmed, extraction of involved teeth may be wise to ensure removal of all the lining in view of the high reported recurrence rate.

Dentigerous cysts contain teeth and, in the young where these are reasonably well placed, treatment may be directed to saving the tooth and allowing it to erupt into the arch.

Cysts may be closely related to the maxillary sinus, floor of nose or to the inferior dental canal, which are important structures not to be damaged and may modify the treatment plan. The maxillary antrum can be partially or even completely obliterated by a large cyst. In the mandible the inferior dental nerve may be grossly displaced in a similar way.

Treatment

Acutely infected cysts are treated with antibacterial drugs and by drainage; further surgery is delayed till the acute phase has settled. There are two methods for treating cysts: enucleation and marsupialisation.

Enucleation

In this operation the whole of the cyst lining is removed. For this reason, and because healing proceeds more rapidly after this has been done, it is the best treatment, particularly for keratocysts, and should be used whenever possible. Though applicable to all types of cyst it is seldom necessary in treating cysts of eruption and is contraindicated in dentigerous cysts if the enclosed tooth is to be preserved.

Small apical cysts where the tooth is to be retained (apicectomy)

These often resolve or remain static following adequate orthograde root canal treatment. If there is evidence of an enlarging radiolucency, or root canal treatment is mechanically impossible, then removal of the cyst together with the apical third of the root may be indicated. The incision is made round the neck of the affected tooth with one or two vertical incisions diverging into the buccal sulcus. The flap is then reflected to expose the bone over the apex (Fig. 13.2).

The position of the root in the alveolar bone is estimated and the apical third exposed. This may be done with a medium-sized rosehead bur. Bone is then removed to expose the cystic area, taking care to avoid damaging, or even exposing, the roots of neighbouring teeth. The apical third of the root is divided using a No. 5 fissure bur. The anterior part of the root should be cut flush with the alveolar bone but bevelled to allow retrograde access to the root canal (Fig. 13.2).

The cyst lining is then enucleated. This does not mean curettage, but implies a careful, methodical separation of the cyst from bone to remove the lining intact without tearing if possible. Curettes (Mitchell's trimmer) can be used,

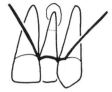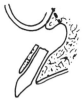

Fig. 13.2 Apicectomy. Left: Apicetomy flap – dotted line shows proposed level of section of root. Right: after root section. Note root cut level with bone margin. Saucerisation may be completed by removing buccal plate to level of dotted line.

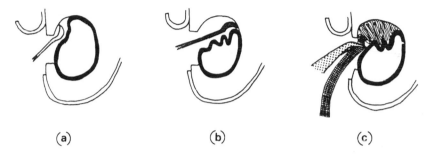

(a)   (b)   (c)

Fig. 13.3 Enucleation of cyst. (a) Curette used to enucleate cyst with the back of the spoon turned towards cyst lining. (b) At greatest diameter of cyst the curette is reversed to present concavity of spoon to the cyst lining. (c) Packing wet ribbon gauze between cyst lining and bone to separate them.

if kept well against bone, to dissect out the cyst gently (Fig. 13.3). Where the lining is firmly attached, 1.5 cm ribbon gauze soaked in saline or in diluted hydrogen peroxide may be packed carefully into the cavity to separate the two tissues (Fig. 13.3). The lining is sent for histological examination. The cavity is examined for any remnants of granulations or cyst lining. These are frequently far back behind the root of the tooth and are removed by scraping the bony walls; none must be left if a recurrence is to be avoided. Where the tooth has been root filled the apical seal is checked. Should this be inadequate a retrograde filling is placed in the apex. The cavity is thoroughly washed out and the flap replaced and sutured.

Where a prosthetic crown is present it is unwise to incise around the gingival margin and a semi-lunar incision 3 cm long is made with its lowest point at least 0.5 cm above the gingival margin. Care must be taken when removing bone to ensure that at the end of the operation the flap margin is adequately supported on bone.

Enucleation of the larger odontogenic cysts

The chief problems in the treatment of large cysts by enucleation are to provide a flap which will give adequate closure and to establish the maximum amount of clot that will organise without liquefying or becoming infected. When these objects are achieved the cyst will heal by first intention with minimal deformity.

Flap

The incision is made at the cervical margin of the teeth or along the alveolar crest in edentulous patients. The design should ensure that at closure the margins are on sound bone and thus it should be adequately extended to allow for the extraction of teeth that might become necessary during the procedure. An envelope flap or three sided design is suitable for most situations (see Chapter 8). Where the bone resorption has brought cyst lining and mucoperiosteum into apposition the two should be separated without tearing either, and the flap reflected beyond the cyst lining on to bone. This is usually the most difficult part of the operation.

Bone removal

It may be possible to peel thin layers of bone from the cyst lining if this is sufficiently thin, but some bone must usually be removed with burs to allow full access to the cavity. The alveolar ridge should be spared as much as possible in order to facilitate the wearing of dentures. Any tooth with a poor prognosis should be removed. If it is in close relation to the lining it should accompany the rest of the specimen for histological examination.

Enucleation

The whole of the cyst lining must be enucleated. After its removal it is carefully examined for any tears or deficiencies. Only where it is intact can the surgeon be sure no lining has been left behind. The cavity is systematically searched and any soft tissue remnants curetted out. This is particularly important where a keratocyst is suspected. The bone edges are saucerised to provide a smooth transition from cyst cavity to the surface of the bone (Figs. 13.4, 13.5 and 13.6). Saucerisation can be extensive providing that the alveolar crest is preserved to leave a satisfactory ridge for dentures and that vital structures are not damaged. Anteriorly the bony support to the ala of the nose must not be undermined lest an ugly deformity occur.

Closure

This needs to be done with care to achieve the elimination of as much dead space as possible. In addition there should a good seal around the margin of the cyst cavity. Post-operative bleeding will cause bulging of the flap and may contribute to breakdown of the wound. A small quantity of a haemostatic agent such as oxidised cellulose may be employed to prevent this. The flap should be encouraged to lie in close apposition to the cyst cavity and mat-

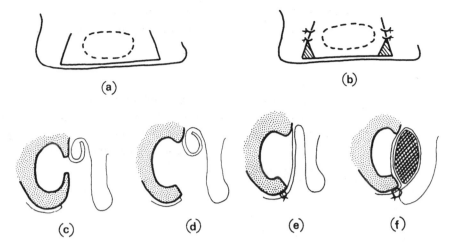

Fig. 13.4 Enucleation of large dental cysts. (a) Section of cyst cavity before saucerisation. (b) After saucerisation. (c) Flap replaced.

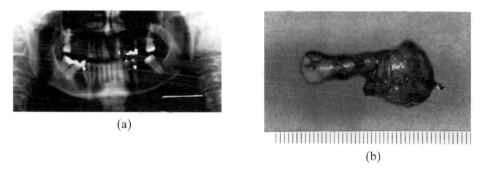

Fig. 13.5 Dental or radicular cyst: (a) Radiographic appearance (b) Following removal; note association with apex of premolar.

tress sutures may help. Added support may be given by an external pressure dressing, particularly in the lower anterior region. This can be removed after 48 hours or when post-operative haemorrhage has ceased. Alternatively, the clot may be reduced by adequate drainage. For cysts in the mandible a drain can be placed from the cavity through the lingual wall below the floor of the mouth and brought out onto the skin of the neck. The drain is removed after 48 hours.

Various substances have been packed into the cyst cavity to obliterate the dead space. Fibrin foam and gelatine sponge only form a matrix for a large clot, which may still become infected. The use of bone is more rational and chips

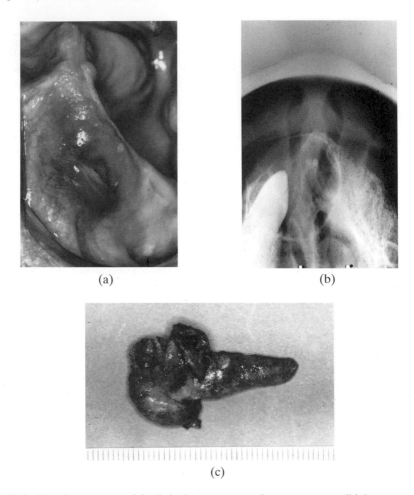

(a)   (b)

(c)

Fig. 13.6 Dentigerous cyst: (a) clinical appearance; denture trauma; (b) large radiolucency associated with crown of unerupted canine; (c) following removal.

have been successfully employed, but also carry a risk of infection. Rarely, in very large cysts of the mandible, the bone can be so weakened at operation that it may be necessary to place an immediate bone graft in the cavity.

Wound breakdown

If the wound should break down the cavity will become contaminated with saliva and food debris. In this event the cavity should be gently packed with $\frac{1}{2}$ in ribbon gauze soaked in Whitehead's varnish, an iodoform preparation, to maintain an antiseptic occlusion of the space for up to 3 weeks. After this time the pack should be changed at intervals until epithelialisation of the wound has occurred. The patient may then be furnished with a syringe to keep the cavity clean. Healing even under these circumstances is remarkably rapid.

Marsupialisation

An opening into the cyst is made so that the contents drain out and the lining epithelium is exposed to the mouth. The advantages of marsupialisation are simplicity, speed of operation, minimal trauma and that no bone is exposed to contamination from the mouth. This makes it ideal for ill patients unable to undergo a long procedure or a general anaesthetic. Marsupialisation lessens the danger of damaging vital structures, the alveolar ridge is preserved and indeed, if properly planned, the operation may improve the depth of the buccal sulcus and the retention of dentures, particularly in the lower jaw. It has two major disadvantages: pathological tissues are left and healing is slow. It should be the treatment of choice only for eruption cysts and dentigerous cysts where the tooth is to be preserved. In large cysts where the jaw may fracture or vital structures, particularly teeth, could be damaged by enucleation, marsupialisation may be used as a first procedure. Once bone has reformed the remaining lining is enucleated at a second operation. This technique has also been successfully used for large keratocysts of the ascending ramus where because the lining is in contact with periosteum over a wide area and dissection is difficult there is a danger of seeding into the soft tissues. Even in this group of cysts new bone appears to reform and make later enucleation safe.

Operation

A buccal incision is made along the occlusal margin of the cyst and curved at each end to follow its contour in the bone. The flap should be large. Some operators make a small hole which tends to close and requires packing over a long period because a satisfactory obturator cannot be fitted. It must be accepted that where many natural teeth are present only a small opening can be made.

The flap is then reflected and the bone removed as widely as possible over the cyst. A window which closely follows the bone margins is cut in the lining with scissors. This tissue should be sent for histological examination. The mucosal flap is now excised so that cyst lining and mucosa can be sewn together round the edges of the window (Fig. 13.7). The cavity is washed out and temporarily dressed with Whitehead's varnish or bismuth, iodoform paraffin paste (BIPP) on ribbon gauze. With a large window in an edentulous area the pack and sutures may be removed after 10 days and an obturator constructed on a denture. The patient is given a water syringe to keep the cavity clean. As the cavity obliterates the obturator will require reduction. Where the aperture is small and an obturator cannot be worn, packing must continue until healing is complete. In dentigerous cysts containing an erupting tooth the same procedure is followed, care being taken not to disturb the tooth (Fig. 13.8).

Marsupialisation into the antrum

Large cysts which encroach on the maxillary antrum can be marsupialised into it. This avoids a gross deformity in the buccal sulcus which may take a long time

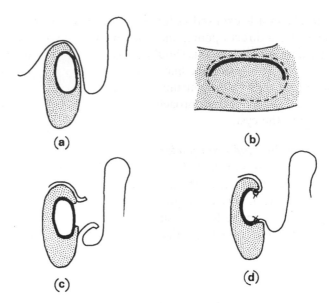

(a)

(b)

(c)

(d)

Fig. 13.7   Marsupialisation. (a) The pre-operative outline of cyst in mandible. (b) Black line shows line of incision in buccal mucoperiosteum and following the outline of the cyst (dotted line). (c) Removal of buccal bone to expose cyst but preserve the alveolar ridge. (d) Cyst opened, drained, and lining sutured to mucous membrane.

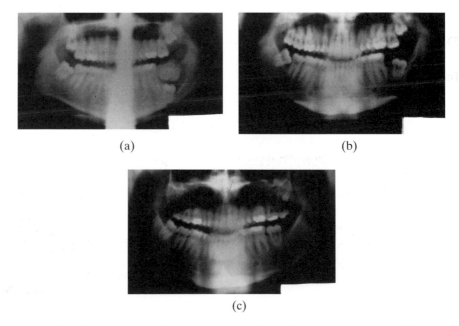

(a)

(b)

(c)

Fig. 13.8   Dentigerous cyst: (a) obstructed eruption of lower second molar; (b) movement of tooth following marsupialisation; (c) eruption of tooth into function.

to heal. The cyst is exposed as for enucleation and a window cut in the lining. Through this a direct opening into the antrum is made where cyst and antrum lining are in apposition. This should be as large as possible and never less than 2.5 cm across. This technique may be combined with enucleation of cysts which are adherent only to the antrum lining. The operation can also be performed through a Caldwell–Luc approach into the antrum when a hole is cut from the antrum into the cyst.

Combined enucleation and open packing

Large cysts can be enucleated, but instead of an immediate closure the mucosal flap is turned into the cavity to cover some of the raw bone and a pack is inserted to protect the rest. This technique overcomes the risk of breakdown of the blood clot present in immediate closure. As the pathological lining has all been removed, healing is far faster than when the cavity is marsupialised.

Follow-up

Long-term follow-up of all cysts is advisable lest retained epithelial fragments cause a recurrence. Satisfactory healing can be assessed by clinical examination, and by radiopaque lamina round the periphery of the cyst and new bone formation filling the radiolucent area.

Keratocysts may recur a long time after operation; follow-up of these lesions must continue over a long period of years.

Developmental cysts of non-dental origin

Inclusion or fissural cysts of the jaws

These arise from the inclusion of epithelial remnants at the site of fusion of the various processes that form the mouth and face. They are epithelial lined and

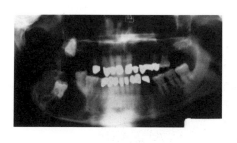

(a)

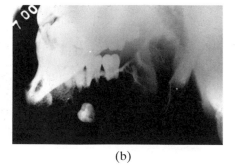

(b)

Fig. 13.9 Diagnostic difficulties: (a) Histologically this lesion was a dental cyst; (b) this lesion was an ameloblastoma.

usually contain mucoid fluid. As they do not arise from the teeth, vitality testing is essential in the differential diagnosis.

Nasolabial cysts

These occur at the junction of the globular, lateral and median nasal processes, under the ala of the nose. They are diagnosed by their position as they lie in a depression on the maxilla, and not in the bone.

Median cysts

These very rare cysts are found in the midline where fusion of the two halves of the palate and mandible takes place.

Incisive canal cysts

These develop from epithelial remnants in the incisive canal. They present as a swelling under the incisive papilla which, on an anterior occlusal radiograph, shows as an expansion of the incisive foramen. The latter is normally under 7 mm in diameter. Occasionally the presenting symptom is a complaint of a salty taste.

Globulomaxillary cysts

These occur at the junction of the globular and maxillary processes. They arise between the maxillary lateral incisor and canine, characteristically separating the roots of these teeth which are not concerned with the formation of the cyst and should be vital.

Diagnosis and assessment

This is approached in the same way as for cysts of dental origin and the differential diagnosis is made by their special features. These are their site, fluid contents, and the fact that adjacent teeth are vital because the cysts are of non-dental origin.

Treatment

They are treated like other cysts of the jaws by enucleation, or by marsupialisation followed by enucleation where there is risk of damaging adjacent teeth.

Non-epithelial lined cysts

Solitary bone cyst

These so-called traumatic bone cysts occur in the jaws, usually in the tooth bearing area. However, they are not associated with dental pathology and

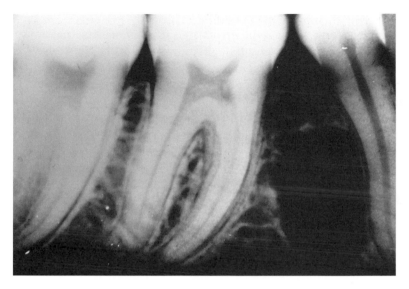

Fig. 13.10 Solitary (traumatic) bone cyst.

are discovered purely on routine radiography. On opening the cyst cavity, little or no lining or contents are found. Any lining present is connective tissue rather than epithelium. They heal spontaneously following light curotage (Fig. 13.10).

Soft tissue cysts

Dermoid cysts

These arise from inclusion of ectoderm at lines of fusion anywhere in the body. In the mouth they may be found in the floor, the palate or the tongue. They are teratomas lined by stratified squamous epithelium and may contain hair, nails, teeth, etc.

Diagnosis

Those in the floor of the mouth may occur in the midline or laterally. They do not become obvious until adolescence or later. The patient complains of a slowly enlarging swelling under the tongue, occasionally affecting speech, and which is visible in the neck. Examination reveals a fluctuant or soft swelling in the floor of the mouth either above or below the mylohyoid. It does not move up or down on swallowing, which is important in distinguishing it from a thyroglossal cyst. Aspiration produces a thick sebaceous material, where this can be withdrawn. Dermoid cysts at other sites are similarly diagnosed.

Treatment

Sublingual dermoids may be enucleated through an external approach below the mandible or intraorally though an incision in the floor of the mouth, just at the reflection of the lingual mucosa from the mandible. The latter flap is reflected lingually and will contain the ducts of the submandibular glands which must not be damaged. The cyst is then exposed but may have to be emptied to remove it as otherwise it may be too large to pass out of the incision. Its thick lining makes it easy to enucleate. Satisfactory drainage must be provided for a few days for the large sublingual deficiency.

Salivary cysts (mucocele)

There are discussed under diseases of the salivary glands (Chapter 16).

Further reading

Cawson, R.A., Langdon, J.D. & Eveson, J.W. (1996) *Surgical Pathology of the Mouth and Jaws*. Wright, Oxford.

Moore, J.R. (1986) *Surgery of the Mouth and Jaws*. Blackwell Scientific Publications, Oxford.

Soames, J.V. & Southam, J.C. (1993) *Oral Pathology*, 2nd edn. Oxford University Press, Oxford.

Chapter 14
Management of Maxillofacial Trauma

- Initial assessment
- Applied anatomy
- Diagnosis
- Treatment planning
- Principles of treatment
- Definitive treatment
- Complications of fractures

The commonest causes of fractured jaws are fights, road accidents, falls and sport. They occur chiefly in males between 15 and 35 years of age and twice as frequently in the mandible as in the maxilla. Fractures may be direct, following a blow at the point where the break occurs, or may be indirect as a result of a blow on the bone at some distance from where the lesion occurs. They may be single, linear or comminuted, that is fragmented into two or more small pieces, and are said to be compound when they communicate with a wound in the skin or mucous membrane of the mouth, nose or air sinuses. Where there is a tooth in the line of the fracture the latter is almost certainly compound into the mouth through the periodontal membrane. In the young, incomplete or greenstick fractures of the mandible can occur. Diseases of the bone predispose to spontaneous pathological fractures. All traumatised patients need to be fully assessed.

Initial assessment

The American College of Surgeons has established a pattern of assessment of the traumatised patient that has been adopted as the gold standard in many countries around the world. This is disseminated through advanced trauma life support courses (ATLS). The initial assessment should not concentrate on the most obvious injury but involve a rapid survey of the vital functions to allow management priorities to be established. The primary survey involves:

- A – Airway maintenance with cervical spine control
- B – Breathing and ventilation
- C – Circulation with haemorrhage control

- D – Disability: neurological status
- E – Exposure: complete examination of the patient

During the primary survey, resuscitation is performed and afterwards shock management is initiated with fluid replacement whilst the vital signs are monitored for any deterioration in the status of the patient.

Once the patient is stabilised a secondary survey is carried out to ensure that all traumatic injuries are evaluated, after which definitive care can be prioritised.

Airway and cervical spine

In unconscious patients respiratory obstruction may be caused by blood clot, or a foreign body in the oropharynx or larynx. In bilateral fractures of the mandible through the canine region the tongue may fall back to occlude the airway. In maxillary injuries the palate can be displaced down and back to occlude the pharynx. Cervical spine injury should be suspected in any blunt trauma above the clavicle and excluded by appropriate radiographs. Until then a hard cervical collar should be worn.

Control of the airway is an absolute priority. The tongue or palate is drawn forward and the mouth and pharynx sucked or wiped clear of debris to re-establish the airway. To keep the tongue forward, a suture may be passed through it, or the patient turned on his side, with control of the cervical spine, to allow saliva and blood to drain out of the mouth. Where these measures are ineffective intubation may be necessary. Before giving an anaesthetic in the unconscious patient soon after the accident the stomach must be emptied of swallowed blood using an orogastric tube.

Haemorrhage

Acute bleeding, though seldom of long duration, is controlled as described in Chapter 7. Reduction and fixation will often arrest haemorrhage because movement disturbs the natural arrest. The pulse and blood pressure should be monitored to ensure that the patient does not become shocked, and appropriate fluid replacement should be started where necessary.

Head injury

Many patients who sustain facial injuries may also have lost consciousness. All these patients, however short the time they were unconscious, must be fully assessed using the Glasgow Coma Scale (GCS) and referred to a neurosurgeon. The Glasgow Coma Scale consists of ranking of behavioural responses (Table 14.1). Motor responses, verbal reponses, and eye opening are independently assessed and scored numerically out of a total of 15. The patient's condition must be carefully observed and recorded for changes in pulse, blood pressure and pupil reaction to light, as these reflect changes in intracranial pressure. A rise in intra-cranial pressure is denoted by a slow reaction to light

Table 14.1   Glasgow coma scale (GCS). Take the best score from each category to give a total coma score.

Eye opening		Motor		Verbal	
Spontaneous	4	moves to command	6	converses	5
To speech	3	localises to pain	5	confused	4
To pain	2	withdraws from pain	4	gibberish	3
None	1	flexes	3	grunts	2
		extends	2	none	1
		none	1		

on the affected side and as the pressure increases the pupil becomes fixed and dilated. As the condition of the patient worsens the opposite pupil also dilates. In the initial stages of assessment and resuscitation following acute trauma, monitoring may be virtually continous but should be maintained even in the apparently stable patient at intervals up to one hourly for 24 hours after the initial trauma.

Prevention of infection

External wounds are kept covered with dressings and a prophylactic course of antibacterial drug is administered. The wounds should be closed as soon as possible, under local anaesthesia if necessary.

Pain

This can be severe particularly with comminuted and grossly displaced fractures, but can sometimes be less than anticipated. Morphine or its derivatives must not be given because they may mask the signs of increasing intracranial pressure, or depress the patient with an embarrassed airway. Non-steroidal anti-inflammatory drugs may be prescribed.

Temporary immobilisation

This has mainly fallen into disuse as early reduction and fixation is to be preferred. However, the use of a barrel bandage to support the comminuted mandible may be advocated. Careful consideration must be given to the effect this may have on the fragments as an ill-applied bandage may increase the displacement.

Supportive treatment

This has been discussed in Chapters 2 and 4.

The management of maxillofacial injuries will now be considered.

Applied anatomy

For describing injuries the face is divided into three parts. The lower third is the mandible and the soft tissues covering it. The middle third is bounded below by the occlusal line of the maxillary teeth and above by a line drawn through the pupils. The upper third lies above this.

The mandible

The commonest sites of fracture in the mandible are the condyle neck, the angle and the canine region. The condyle may fracture through its thin neck either within the capsule or below it, and may be bilateral as a result of blows to the chin, particularly if the mouth is open, or unilateral following blows to the body of the mandible on the opposite side. Fractures of the coronoid process are uncommon.

The angle of the mandible is a weak point because there is a change in the direction of the grain of the bone which occurs where the vertical ascending ramus and horizontal body meet. Further, the shape of the mandible in cross-section changes as the thick lower border of the body becomes thin at the angle, so that the lower third molar sits in bone with little basal support lingually. Finally, the third molar, particularly if it is unerupted, may occupy up to two-thirds of the depth of the bone.

The body is the strongest part of the lower jaw but is weakened by the presence of the tooth sockets. The canine has a long broad root and its socket is a common site of fracture. The symphysis may also be involved as a result of blows on the chin. Alveolar fractures occur chiefly in the incisor region.

Displacement

Displacement depends on three factors, the force of the blow, gravity and the pull of the muscles inserted into the bone. The muscles concerned are the suprahyoid group attached to the lingual aspect of the anterior part of the mandible which depress the lower jaw, and the muscles of mastication (masseter, temporalis and medial pterygoid) inserted into the ascending ramus which elevate the mandible and move it laterally. The lateral pterygoid muscle, inserted into the condyle and meniscus of the temporomandibular joint, draws the condyle forward and therefore assists in opening the mouth.

Condylar fractures

In these cases the lateral pterygoid muscle draws the fractured head forward medially and, in certain cases, over the eminentia articularis and out of the glenoid fossa to produce a fracture dislocation. The other muscles of mastication raise the ramus of the affected side to produce an anterior open bite between the incisors and canines on the opposite side. On opening the mouth

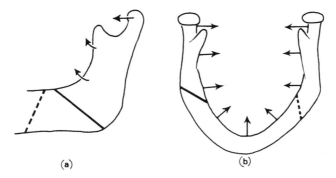

Fig. 14.1   Effects of muscle pull on mandibular fractures. Arrows indicate the direction of muscle pull. (a) Horizontal view of mandible showing horizontally favourable fracture (dotted line) and horizontally unfavourable fracture (continuous line), (b) Vertical view showing vertically favourable (dotted line) and unfavourable (continuous line) fractures.

the body of the mandible is displaced towards the affected side with marked deviation of the midline. In bilateral condylar fractures both ascending rami are drawn up and back equally so that gagging occurs on the posterior teeth causing an anterior open bite on both sides.

Fractures of the angle or body

In these the suprahyoid group of muscles depress the anterior part of the mandible. Posteriorly the pull of the muscles of mastication attached to the ascending ramus draws it upwards. The posterior fragment is also drawn inwards as the pull of the medial pterygoid muscle is stronger than that of the masseter (Fig. 14.1). Displacement is resisted by the periosteum, if it is intact, by the occlusion of the teeth, and by the impaction of the fractured bone ends against each other. This last depends on the angle of the line of fracture which is said to be *unfavourable* if it would allow the posterior fragment to displace or *favourable* if it prevents it doing so.

As displacement can take place in two planes, upwards and inwards, fractures are described as favourable or unfavourable when viewed from the side or horizontally, and from above or vertically. Thus a horizontally unfavourable fracture displaces upwards, a vertically unfavourable fracture inwards (Fig. 14.1).

Where a bilateral fracture occurs in the anterior region through the canine sockets it is possible for the geniohyoid, genioglossus and mylohyoid muscles to displace the loose anterior portion downwards and backwards, with loss of control of the tongue which may fall back into the pharynx and obstruct the airway.

Midline fracture

In oblique fractures through the symphysis of the mandible, one half may be displaced lingually by the mylohyoid muscle to cause over-riding in the midline.

Age

In children the mandible is greatly weakened by the numerous crypts of the developing teeth but the greater elasticity of the bone compensates for this. In older patients the bones get more brittle and tend to break more easily and the mandible is weakened by resorption of the alveolar bone after the teeth are lost. The periosteum does however form a complete envelope round the edentulous mandible which, if not torn in the accident, holds the fractured ends in apposition. With advancing years the mandible becomes more dependent for its blood supply on the periosteum than on the inferior dental artery. For this reason methods of reduction or fixation which involve stripping of the periosteum must be avoided in the elderly.

Middle third of the face

Fractures of the middle third of the face involve a complex of bones which include the paired bones, the maxilla, palatine, zygomatic, nasal, lachrymal and inferior conchae, together with the single vomer and ethmoid bones. The structure of the maxillary complex consists of a grid system of buttresses (Fig. 14.2).

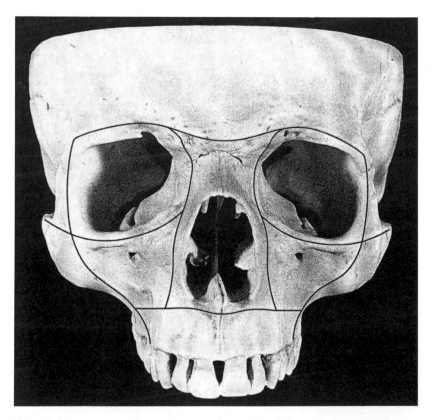

Fig. 14.2 Grid structure of face: these are the principal lines of reconstruction.

Strong vertical buttresses are formed by the frontal process of the maxilla, the zygomatic process of the maxilla and the zygomatic bone, and the pterygoid plates of the sphenoid with the tuberosity of the maxilla. Horizontal buttresses are formed by the supraorbital margin, the infraorbital margin, and the palatine bones in continuity with the alveolar process. The spaces between are closed with thin bone plates which enclose several large cavities, the maxillary air sinuses, the nasal cavity and the orbits. The vertical buttresses are more functionally challenged through the forces of mastication, particularly in the first permanent molar and canine regions, and the middle third is thus more resistant to upward forces but less to shearing stress from a horizontal blow.

Fractures of the middle third of the face fall into six categories (Fig. 14.3):

- Alveolar
- Guerin's/Le Fort I
- Pyramidal/Le Fort II
- High transverse/Le Fort III

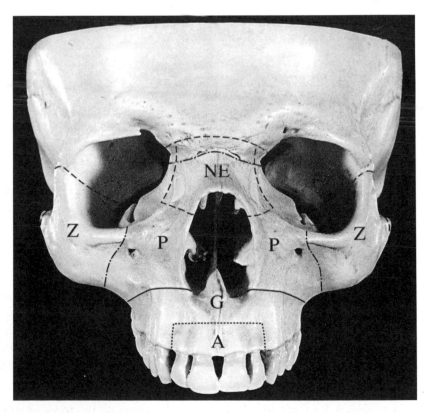

Fig. 14.3 Fractures of the mid-third of the face: A – alveolar; G – Guerin's (Le Fort I); P – Pyramidal (Le Fort II); Z – zygomatic (malar); NE – naso-ethmoidal; Le Fort III is shown by the upper dotted line.

- Naso-ethmoidal complex
- Malar/zygomatic

Alveolar fractures

Alveolar fractures occur in the tooth bearing areas of the jaw.

Guerin's or Le Fort I fractures

These occur where the palate and alveolus are separated from the maxillary complex by a transverse fracture just above the floor of the nose and the antrum.

Pyramidal or Le Fort II fracture

The fracture line passes through the lateral and anterior walls of the maxillary sinuses and continues up through the infraorbital margins to join across the bridge of the nose.

High transverse or Le Fort III

The maxillary complex is virtually separated from the cranium by a fracture which traverses the lateral walls of both orbits and both orbital floors and crosses the midline at the root of the nose to involve the cribriform plate of the ethmoid.

The nasal bones and naso-ethmoidal complex

This may be involved separately or in combination with other fractures.

The malar bone (zygoma)

This can be fractured by a direct blow which may drive in the prominence of the cheek. The fracture line passes through the infraorbital margin, the anterior wall of the antrum, the malar buttress, the zygomatic arch and the frontal process of the zygoma.

The clinical importance of this classification is that the Le Fort I involves only the palate and maxillary antrum. The Le Fort II involves the antrum, floor of the orbit and the nose. The Le Fort III includes the structures affected by the Le Fort II and also the anterior cranial fossa. It is emphasised that all Le Fort III fractures are head injuries and should be monitored as such. Further, as the anterior cranial fossa communicates with the nose through the fractured cribriform plate there is a grave danger of an ascending infection. The patient must be protected from a meningeal infection by the prescription of appropriate antibiotics. A cerebrospinal fluid leak may require an intracranial dural repair by neurosurgeons which may be effected at the same time as fracture fixation. Thus the management of such injuries calls for a team approach.

Displacement

In maxillary fractures the displacement is caused by the force of the blow and not by muscle pull as none of the muscles attached to the maxilla are strong enough to move the fragments. The most usual displacement is backwards and downwards, causing a typical concavity of the face (dish-face) with anterior open bite due to gagging on the posterior teeth. This open bite is particularly marked in the Guerin's type fracture.

Diagnosis

The oral surgeon should proceed to make a diagnosis in the usual way unless some urgent condition identified in the primary survey requires immediate attention.

History

The time of the accident is important in assessing the urgency of treatment, and the degree of infection in compound fractures. The difficulty of reducing misplaced fractures increases as healing progresses. A history of any previous facial injury is important as old injuries can occasionally cause confusion in the diagnosis. The patient's general condition and any tenderness or bruising of the head, chest or abdomen are noted. Shock is unusual in facial injuries and, unless the blood loss has been excessive, the cause should be sought elsewhere.

The patient should be asked if he was knocked out. In unconscious or confused patients causes other than concussion such as alcohol, recreational drugs, insulin or diabetic coma, or a cardiovascular catastrophe should be considered. Any drug administered previously, especially sedatives, analgesics or antibacterials, should be recorded.

Examination

The surgeon must consider all the possible tissues that might be involved in the trauma – skin, connective tissue, blood vessels, nerves (both sensory and motor), muscles, underlying bones – together with special structures such as the eyes and salivary glands. The following signs of a fracture must be looked for. Swelling and bruising are usual at the point where the patient was struck, but may not coincide with the site of an indirect fracture. Deformity of the bone contour can be masked by swelling, but examination may reveal a break in the continuity of the bone or displacement. Intraorally derangement of the occlusion may localise the fracture. Abnormal movement in the bone is diagnostic and when it occurs may be accompanied by pain and by crepitus or grating as the rough bone ends rub against each other. Loss of function in the jaws is common as a result of trismus or pain.

The facial bones can be conveniently examined in the dental chair but should the patient be too ill to get out of bed the headboard may be removed to allow the patient to be examined from above and behind.

Extraoral

The patient is first looked at full face for obvious signs of injury. Lacerations should not be probed or touched but are immediately covered with a dressing, Clots present in the nose and ears should not be disturbed but a discharge of cerebrospinal fluid (CSF) from these orifices is an important finding indicating a fracture of the cranial base. To distinguish it from nasal secretion it should be tested for glucose, a constituent of CSF. CSF in contradistinction to blood does not clot and this can usefully differentiate them.

The surgeon should then move behind the patient and, looking down from above, he uses the tips of his fingers to palpate and compare the right and left sides, and to determine points of tenderness or breaks in the continuity of the facial bones. He starts with the superior, lateral and inferior margins of the orbit and then proceeds to the bridge of the nose, where any deviation from the midline or depression is noted. The malar prominences are compared to detect loss of contour. Where there is marked oedema if may be very difficult to do this with certainty, but firm steady pressure on the swelling for a few moments will push it away and allow the bone to be felt.

The fingers then move over the zygomatic arch, to the temporomandibular joints. The patient is asked to open and close the mouth and perform lateral movements. The range of opening and of lateral movement is assessed. Fractures of the zygomatic arch may prevent opening as the coronoid process may jam against the displaced zygomatic process. In fractures of the condyle or ascending ramus there is little movement of the condyle head on the affected side or the mandible towards the opposite side. When the joint is difficult to palpate the little finger may be put into the external auditory meatus and the condyle felt through the anterior wall. Palpation is then continued to compare the ascending ramus, the angles and the lower border of the body of the mandible.

The surgeon then moves to face the patient and examines the eyes for damage, particularly depression, proptosis or a difference in level. The intercanthal distance should be measured from the midline. Any difference in the values on either side or a marked increase from the normal range suggests a traumatic detachment of the medial canthal ligaments. Subconjunctival haemorrhage without posterior limit in the upper half of the eye suggests bleeding from a fracture of the roof of the orbit, and in the lower part of the conjunctiva a fracture of the orbital floor, but in severe injuries the whole of the conjunctiva may be involved. Each eye is checked individually for vision and then both together for movement vertically and horizontally and for double vision (diplopia) in all fields. This can be done by moving a finger up, down and across where it can be clearly seen by both eyes at once. Abnormalities of movement and diplopia may be due to paralysis of the extrinsic muscles of the eye as a result of cranial injury. Diplopia alone may be caused by detachment of the suspensory ligament in malar or maxillary fractures, herniation of orbital fat through defects in the orbital floor, or by oedema, all of which may alter the position of the eyeball. Oedema can also mask diplopia by compensating for a fall in level which may only become apparent when the swelling recedes. Visual acuity should also be tested in the conscious patient. The examination concludes with tests for loss of sensation in the branches of the trigeminal nerve, particularly the infraorbital, which is affected in malar and maxillary fractures, and the mental nerve involved in mandibular injuries. Function of the facial nerve is checked by asking the patient to move his forehead, eyelids and lips.

Intraoral

The lips are gently parted and the mucosa, floor of the mouth and tongue examined for lacerations or haematoma. A haematoma of the floor of the mouth is a sign of a fracture of the mandible. The teeth are charted and those that are lost, grossly carious or fractured are noted, together with any disturbance of the occlusion. Where teeth (or denture fragments) are missing and cannot be accounted for, particularly if the patient has lost consciousness, the chest should be radiographed. Percussion of the teeth may give a 'cracked teacup' note suggestive of a broken tooth or of a fractured jaw, particularly in the maxilla. The upper buccal sulcus is palpated for any sharp edges of bone or bruising diagnostic of a fracture through the malar buttress.

Fractures of the maxillary alveolus or a midline split of the palate are detected by grasping the alveolar segments and trying gently at first to move them by grasping the alveolus and the teeth in one hand and trying to elicit movement, whilst the other hand palpates extraorally to determine the level at which the fracture has occurred. The fingers are placed in turn over the root of the nose, at the infraorbital margins and in the canine fossa.

Similarly the mandible is grasped in both hands, with the fingers over the occlusal surface of the teeth and the thumbs under the lower border, and tested in segments for mobility. The clinical findings should be written down and a provisional diagnosis made before radiographs are ordered.

A summary of the diagnostic features of various fractures is shown in Table 14.2.

Radiographs

Radiographs are taken to establish the presence of fractures, the direction in which they run and the amount by which they are displaced, and to identify radiopaque foreign bodies such as glass in the soft tissues. Medicolegally they are considered a diagnostic measure of the first importance. They also provide a visual record of the progress of the patient.

Radiographs of all fractures must be taken in two planes. The following views usually give a satisfactory survey of the facial bones and wherever there is doubt about the extent of the injuries all should be taken. They are a dental panoramic

Table 14.2   Diagnostic features of fractures. All these signs and symptoms are not found in every case. Radiographs will show a lack of continuity in the bone at the site of the fracture.

Site	Signs and symptoms
Unilateral condyle	Affected side: Pain in joint, worse on moving Tenderness and swelling Absence (or abnormality) of movements of condyle head Deviation of mandible towards this side Gagging on molar teeth Opposite side: open bite Limitation of lateral excursion to that side
Bilateral condyle	Pain, tenderness and swelling over both joints Gagging on the posterior teeth and an anterior open bite Restricted lateral movements Absence of movement of condyle heads
Body of the mandible	Pain on moving jaw Trismus Movement and crepitus at site of fracture Step deformity of lower border of mandible Derangement of the occlusion Mental anaesthesia Haematoma in the floor of mouth and buccal mucosa
Malar	Depression of the prominence of the cheek Step deformity in the infraorbital ridge Subconjunctival haemorrhage and diplopia Infraorbital nerve anaesthesia Haematoma intraorally over the malar buttress Blood in the antrum Trismus due to the coronoid process impacting against the displaced malar or zygomatic arch Circumorbital ecchymosis
Guerin's (Le Fort I)	Floating palate Blood in the antrum Bilateral haematoma in buccal sulcus Deranged occlusion with anterior open bite
Low pyramidal (Le Fort II)	Gross swelling and, after oedema subsides, dish-faced deformity Subconjunctival haemorrhage and diplopia Bilateral infraorbital nerve anaesthesia Bilateral haematoma intraorally over malar buttresses Retroposed upper dental arch with anterior open bite
High transverse (Le Fort III)	Gross swelling and, after oedema subsides, dish-faced deformity Subconjunctival haemorrhage and sometimes diplopia Retroposed upper dental arch with anterior open bite Cerebrospinal fluid leak from nose Signs of head injury

Table 14.3 Facial radiographs in maxillofacial trauma.

Site of injury	Radiographic views	Area visualised
Mandible	DPT, OPT	All areas except lower anterior
	Lateral oblique	Good for angle, body, and condyle
	PA mandible	Shows horizontal displacement at angle and condyles
	Lower occlusal	Anterior region
Zygoma	Occipito-mental (OM) 10°–30°	Orbital margins, malar buttress, antrum
	Submento-vertex	Zygomatic arch, supraorbital margin
	Computerised tomography (CT)	Orbital blowouts
Maxilla	As for zygoma	As above
	Lateral face	Shows backward displacement, pterygoid plates, anterior open bite
	Computerised tomography (CT)	Orbital contour, optic nerve, naso-ethmoidal complex
Naso-ethmoidal complex	Computerised tomography (CT)	Good detail, can get reconstructions from CT

tomograph (DPT or OPT), or if the patient is non-ambulatory lateral oblique views of the mandible can be used instead, a postero-anterior view of the mandible, occipito-mental views of the sinuses (10, 15, or 20°), a submento-vertex, and a true lateral of the facial bones. Note that the midline of the mandible is difficult to see except on an occlusal film. Fractures involving the naso-ethmoidal complex should always be visualised using computerised axial tomography (CT).

Examination of the radiographs is first made to identify all the normal structures and the bony margins of the facial bones. Both sides of the jaws are compared for differences in outline. It is important to recognise shadows thrown by such normal structures as the oropharyngeal airway, hyoid bone or intervertebral spaces, which may simulate fractures in certain projections.

The dental panoramic tomograph (DPT)

This tomographic radiograph of the jaws has largely replaced the lateral oblique views. However, it is unsuitable for any patient who is unable to stand or sit whilst the radiograph is being taken and in this case the latter should be considered. The mandible from condyle to condyle is seen but due to super-imposition of the cervical spine the canine and incisor regions may not be well visualised. As the rotation of the X-ray tube changes direction in the premolar region, caution is needed in interpretation in this area. The principal indication for this view is in the diagnosis of fractured mandibles but some information about the lower part of the middle third can also be gleaned (Fig. 14.4).

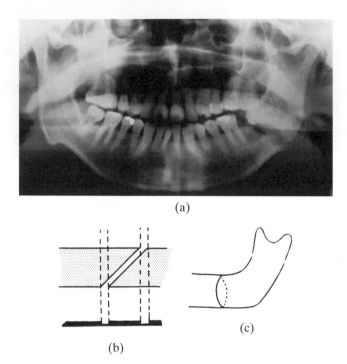

(a)

(b)

(c)

Fig. 14.4 (a) An orthopantomogram showing a displaced fracture of the mandible. Drawing (b) shows how one oblique fracture passing through inner and outer cortical plates may give a false appearance of a double fracture on radiograph. (c) In such a case the fracture lines are always seen to meet at the upper and lower border of the bone.

The postero-anterior view of the mandible

The whole of the mandible from the condyle neck to the midline on both sides is shown. As the rays pass through the angle of the mandible from the lower border to the occlusal surface they give a vertical view of this area and allow vertically favourable and unfavourable fractures to be assessed (Fig. 14.5).

The occipitomental view

This is examined in a series of transverse sweeps following the bony contours at the levels of the supraorbital ridges, of the infraorbital margins, and the zygomatic arch, of the antral wall, nasal wall and vomer, and finally the level of the mandibular/maxillary occlusion and of the lower border of the mandible. It demonstrates fractures of the maxillary complex, and radiopacity of the maxillary sinus which may be the result of bleeding into the antrum from a fracture of one of its walls (Fig. 14.6). Fifteen- or thirty-degree occipito-mental and stereoscopic occipito-mental views are both of assistance in detecting displacement not shown on the standard views. Fractures of the zygomatic arch are best shown on a submentovertex film.

Fig. 14.5   Posterior-anterior view of
mandible showing a vertically favourable
fracture through the angle on the left. A
vertically unfavourable fracture (VU)
may not show on this view as the break in
continuity of the cortical plates may not
be projected on the radiograph. A
vertically favourable fracture (VF) is
usually clearly seen.

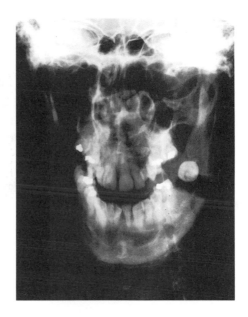

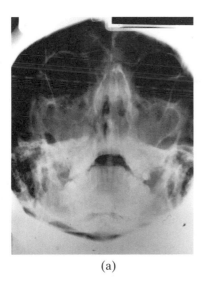

(a)

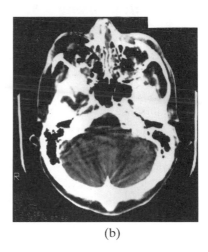

(b)

Fig. 14.6   (a) Occipito-mental view of mid-third trauma showing pan-facial fractures;
(b) CT scan of same patient – note appearance of soft tissue. This patient is seen in
Fig. 14.13.

True lateral of facial bones

This shows separation of the maxilla from the cranial base, or of the palate from
the maxilla, as well as any discontinuity of the pterygoid plates.

Other radiographs of importance are occlusal films and intraoral apical views
of the teeth showing their relationship to the fracture line of their roots. Special

views of the temporomandibular joints may be necessary to show the condyles and the condyle neck.

Computerised axial tomography (CT)

This is now available in most centres and can give valuable information when plain films cannot be taken. The head injured patient is frequently scanned during the initial assessment period and, if it is thought that facial injuries have been sustained, particularly in the mid-face, including this area in the scan can save time in diagnosis. CT is virtually essential in the assessment of naso-ethmoidal injuries and orbital floor trauma. Computed reconstructions of these areas from coronal tomography can be particularly useful.

Study models

Frequently the patient is unable to bring his teeth into occlusion or the fractures are badly comminuted so that the normal relationship of the teeth can only be seen on study models.

Treatment planning

The aims of treatment are to restore function and to achieve a good aesthetic result, but treatment must be modified according to the patient's general condition. The only immediate local measures required are attention to the airway, arrest of haemorrhage and control of infection. Where multiple injuries are present the oral surgeon is responsible for explaining the degree of urgency for treatment of the jaws to achieve a satisfactory result. Thereafter, planning is done jointly with the other specialists involved. It is generally agreed that bony injuries heal better the earlier they are treated but, in the presence of gross oedema or large haematomas, they may be left a few days for these to settle.

Natural repair of bone

The healing of fractures takes place entirely by the natural process of bone repair. Treatment is directed to providing ideal conditions for this to take place.

Between the fractured ends of the bone a blood clot forms. Within four days capillaries, fibroblasts and inflammatory cells invade this and begin replacing it with granulation tissue. Along the bony margins of the fracture osteoclasts appear which resorb the bone; this is seen on radiographs as a widening of the fracture line. Osteoblasts from the periosteum and cancellous bone invade the granulations and lay down a collagenous matrix called osteoid. The acidity of the tissues caused by the initial inflammatory reaction subsides after 10 days and this allows calcification to proceed. Bony union takes place in 4–6 weeks.

The pattern of the new bone or callus is at first irregular but later, over a period of about six months in the mandible, reorganisation to normal bone structure takes place. In long bones an excess of callus is formed round the bone ends, and its presence on radiographs is accepted as a sign that satisfactory union is proceeding. This does not happen in the mandible, where formation of callus is usually limited to the space between the bone ends and therefore shows little on radiographs. Maxillary fractures may heal by fibrous union only.

Principles of treatment

Control of infection

Repair, particularly new bone formation, cannot take place in the presence of infection. To prevent this occurring all foreign bodies, dead bone and tissue are removed from the wound which is then closed to cover the exposed bone. Any movement of bone fractures may predispose to infection and fracture treatment should aim to eliminate this. Antibacterial drugs are administered prophylactically till the inflammatory reaction has resolved and the soft tissue wounds have healed satisfactorily. Drainage is provided if suppuration occurs and causes of infection should be sought and treated as appropriate.

Tooth in the line of fracture

In the jaws the fracture line often passes through a tooth socket leaving one side of the root exposed in the wound. The fracture is then compound into the mouth as tearing of the gingival attachment provides a portal of entry to the mouth organisms. Exposed cementum on the surface of the root rapidly dies and repair may not take place between this inert cementum and new bone, so that healing is delayed. As a result of the accident the pulp may become non-vital and a focus of infection. It is wise, therefore, to extract teeth in the line of fracture where there is gross displacement unless they are to be retained temporarily to establish the occlusion. Where there is little displacement of the fracture the teeth may be kept unless they delay union. The vitality must be checked and non-vital teeth treated as appropriate. In the maxilla vital teeth may be kept, as experience has shown that teeth in the fracture line seldom affect union in the upper jaw.

Reduction of fractures

In reducing fractures the object is to reappose the bone ends as accurately as possible. Although the surgeon should attempt to get perfect reduction the aim is to treat not a radiograph, but a patient, and where displacement is acceptable and function is not impaired the patient should not be subjected to unnecessary surgery.

Perfect reduction may be impossible where there has been gross comminution or tissue loss, and healing will not take place between the fractured ends if the gap is too wide (over 6mm). In comminuted fractures all fragments attached to periosteum must be kept.

The best guide to accurate reduction is the occlusion of the teeth, because of the precise way in which the teeth interdigitate. Further, if the occlusion is restored, masticatory function should be satisfactory. In edentulous patients the dentures are the only sound guide. Where they are lost the site of the accident should be searched or a spare set may be available. The fractured jaw is reduced to the sound jaw, but where many teeth are missing or both jaws badly comminuted, the problem is more difficult. The surgeon must then rely more on anatomical reduction of the bony margins, appearance of the patient, and the results shown on post-operative radiographs.

Reduction should be done as soon as possible but where delay is unavoidable it should be remembered that great difficulty will be experienced in reducing maxillary fractures after 10 days and mandibular fractures after 3 weeks.

Immobilisation of the fragments

Any movement in the fracture line after reduction may disturb or tear the granulations or osteoid tissue. It may also cause the bone to heal with a deformity. Immobilisation should therefore be complete, and continued till union has taken place, which in the mandible is about 4–6 weeks and in the maxilla fibrous union is accepted as 3–4 weeks.

Open reduction and rigid internal fixation (ORIF)

This technique relies on open reduction and rigid fixation of the bone to eliminate movement of the fragments and thus can make further immobilisation unnecessary. It allows uneventful bone healing to occur even under function.

Anaesthesia

Fractures with appreciable displacement are usually reduced under a general anaesthetic. In mandibular fractures a cuffed intranasal endotracheal tube can be passed quite easily despite some pre-operative trismus, but in maxillary fractures involving the cranial base there is often some degree of difficulty and danger in passing a tube through the nose as it may pass into the anterior cranial fossa with disastrous consequences. In this situation an oral tube may suffice if it does not interfere with the occlusion. In the fully dentate patient a submental approach allows an oral tube to be passed through a small submental incision into the floor of the mouth and thus into the larynx. If it is anticipated that more than one surgical intervention is likely then the need for a tracheostomy to provide a safe and efficient anaesthetic must be considered. This may be chosen in the polytraumatised patient in order to maintain respiratory function in those slow to regain consciousness.

Where the jaws are to be fixed together under an anaesthetic, a tongue suture may be employed. This is placed well back to enable the tongue to be drawn forwards out of the pharynx during the recovery period and can be removed once the patient has full control of his airway. The throat pack must be removed prior to the jaws being fixed together. This may best be achieved with elastics which are easily cut with scissors in an emergency but if wires are to be used then the ends should be left long to enable them to be easily identified.

Definitive treatment

Soft tissue repair

All wounds are first carefully explored and foreign bodies and dirt removed. Glass is not easy to find and road or coal dust is difficult to get out but if left gives rise to a tattooed scar. To clear wounds or skin abrasions they are gently scrubbed with water, soap and a soft brush, and thoroughly irrigated.

All tissues about the face are precious and, fortunately, because of their rich blood supply, are very viable. Excision is not practised except on tags of loose, dead skin or mucous membrane or round the edges of wounds that are several days old and may have started to epithelialise. Lacerations are then closed in layers by primary suture, with drains inserted where necessary.

Where there has been loss of skin, the edges must not be drawn together under tension as this leads to deformity and scar formation. Full thickness loss in cheek or lips may be temporarily repaired by sewing skin to mucous membrane. This prevents scarring, protects the deeper tissues and provides a satisfactory base for reconstruction.

Tears in the mucosa must be closed to cover exposed bone. Mucous membrane is easier to manipulate than skin so that by undermining edges and rotating flaps deficiencies can usually be made up.

Where bone and soft tissue surgery are being done at the same operation, soft tissue repair is completed after the fractures have been reduced and fixed.

Mandibular fractures

Intermaxillary fixation (IMF)

The mandible is immobilised by fixing it to the maxilla. This establishes the occlusion and may be a part of the treatment of both mandibular and maxillary fractures. IMF may be achieved in a number of ways.

Temporary

Monocortical bone screws placed between the roots of the canines and premolars in each quadrant can allow IMF to be established during the operative procedure but will not withstand long periods of immobilisation.

Methods using the teeth for fixation

Eyelet wiring

This method is swift, requires no technician or laboratory, and leaves the teeth uncovered so that they can be brought accurately into occlusion. Its

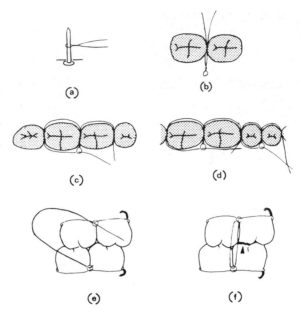

Fig. 14.7 Eyelet wiring. (a) Making eyelet with two twists only of tails. (b) Tails of eyelet wire passed between the teeth from buccal side. (c) Distal wire passed through the eyelet. (d) *Left*, shows correct relationship of wire, flat against the tooth, for twisting. *Right*, incorrect relationship. (e) Intermaxillary wire passed from distal aspect of eyelets. (f) Intermaxillary wires tightened.

disadvantages are that several pairs of sound teeth with a good periodontal condition must be present in each jaw and occlude with similar pairs in the opposite jaw. The eyelet wires are harmless for short periods (6 weeks) but in time they tend to loosen the teeth. Finally, immobilisation is less satisfactory than with arch bars as the wires tend to stretch and loosen.

The eyelet is passed from the buccal side between two adjacent teeth below their contact point and out buccally. The posterior tail is passed through the eyelet (Fig. 14.7) and the two tails are then firmly twisted up. It is important that the wire is drawn tight round the necks of the teeth below the enamel and the first twist is made as close to the tooth as possible (Fig. 14.7). Wires are always twisted clockwise to avoid confusion later when tightening them. Eyelets are put on three or four pairs of teeth as required and on to opposing pairs of teeth in the opposite jaw. Intermaxillary fixation is put in place with a piece of wire passed through corresponding eyelets, and drawn tight and twisted up (Fig. 14.7). All wire ends must be turned into the gum or between the teeth to avoid irritating the mucosa.

Arch bars

These may be more suitable where there are inconvenient gaps in the dental arch which make eyelet wiring impossible. Close fitting cast arch bars may be

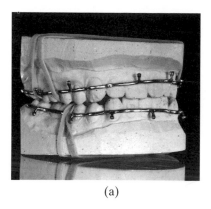
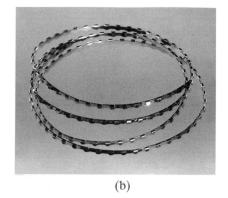

(a)   (b)

Fig. 14.8 Arch bars: (a) custom made arch bars; (b) preformed arch bars can be cut to length from a roll.

constructed from study models if time allows but preformed bars are also available for immediate use (Fig. 14.8). These are bent to fix closely to the teeth in the upper and lower arches while the fractures are held in their reduced position. Wires are passed around the teeth to hold the bar in place. Once the arch bar has been tied across the fracture line further adjustment to the reduction is difficult.

Open reduction and rigid internal fixation (ORIF)

This concept has been accepted as the standard treatment for the vast majority of facial fractures. The technique relies on exposing the fractures through intra- or extraoral incisions and accurate reduction of the bony fractures which are then held rigidly in place by the application of malleable metal plates. This method was originally developed for use in the mandible but is now routinely used to treat all facial fractures. The application of rigid fixation enables bone healing to take place without immobilisation of the bone. Long periods of IMF are thus not necessary and return to function is much more rapid. A well designed plating tool kit integrated with a selection of plate sizes graded by screw diameter (from 2 mm down to 1 mm) provides a flexible system of fixation for all the facial bones (Fig. 14.9).

ORIF of mandibular fractures

Plating of the mandible has the advantage that post-operative intermaxillary fixation is not essential but may be applied whilst the plate is being placed.

Monocortical miniplates

Titanium miniplates are inserted across the fracture line via an intraoral approach. The incision is made through the mucoperiosteum below the attached gingivae with due consideration of vital structures such as the mental nerve. To expose the symphysis region the incision should be flared out into the lip to reduce the chance of wound breakdown. The fracture is identified and reduced

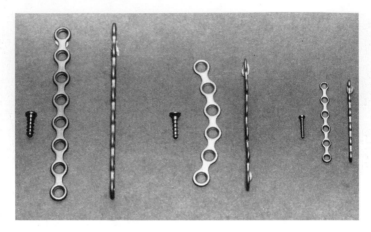

Fig. 14.9   Titanium plates for facial fractures from left: 2.0 mm used in mandibular fractures, 1.7 mm (low profile) and 1.0 mm used in mid-third fractures.

accurately; to effect this any debris in the fracture line should be removed and irrigation performed to allow good visualisation. The occlusion is established and may be maintained by an assistant or by the application of temporary IMF.

Titanium miniplates of 2 mm are standardly used in the fixation of mandibular fractures. It is crucial that the plate is accurately adapted to the contour of the bone and the operator should strive to achieve this. Holes are then drilled through the outer cortical bone to enable monocortical self-tapping titanium screws to be placed. The holes are drilled with burs slightly smaller than the screw diameter to ensure firm screw fixation. The screw should be inserted at the same angle as the drill and advanced slowly through the bone. After each forward turn a reverse turn should be made until the self-tapped hole is established. The screw is then tightened but care should be taken not to strip the threads in the bone. Emergency screws of a greater diameter are available should this arise. Care should be taken to avoid damaging the teeth and suitable screw lengths should be chosen; screws of 7 mm length are standardly used in the mandible. The plate should be selected to allow at least two screws to be placed either side of the fracture. In comminuted fractures longer plates may have to be used in order to achieve this but four hole plates suffice in most situations. In the anterior region of the mandible two plates are placed across the fracture to counteract increased torsional forces, whilst in the body and angle one plate only may be needed (Fig. 14.10). Titanium is a bio-inert material and thus plates do not have to be removed unless they become exposed or the patient becomes aware of them. If rigid fixation is achieved bone healing will take place even in the presence of infection.

Bicortical plates

More rigid plates in conjunction with screws that engage both cortices of the bone are available; these must be placed at the lower border of the mandible

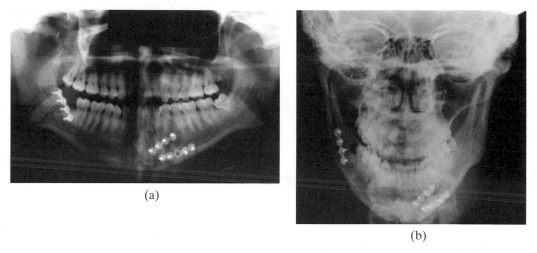

(a)

(b)

Fig. 14.10   Plating of mandibular fractures – note two plates at parasymphysis and one at angle: (a) orthopantomogram; (b) Posterior-anterior view of same patient.

in order to avoid traumatising the teeth. As this often requires an extraoral approach these plates are most frequently used when loss of bone from the fracture site has occurred.

Condylar fractures

The fractured condyle head is usually displaced forward and medially by the lateral pterygoid muscle, while the muscles of mastication tend to draw the ascending ramus up and back to produce an open bite, with rotation of the symphysis menti towards the affected side. Reduction is directed to correcting the displacement of the mandible only. This many patients can be taught to do, using their hands at first to assist in re-educating the muscles of mastication. The patient should be told to stay on a soft diet and analgesics should be prescribed. Where swelling and pain make this difficult, IMF may be applied for 1–2 weeks using arch bars and elastics to encourage the re-establishment of the occlusion. In fracture dislocations the same treatment is adequate as it has been shown that, though union occurs in an abnormal position, the head of the condyle remodels to make a functional joint. Where other mandibular fractures are present these should be treated as indicated and the need for IMF assessed following this.

Bilateral condylar fractures

The management of bilateral condylar fractures is complicated due to an increased incidence of anterior open bite and this does not always respond to a period of IMF. Open reduction and internal fixation of at least one of the fractured condyles may be indicated if these fractures lie outside the joint capsule. This particularly applies in panfacial fractures where the spacial geometry of the face may be difficult to reconstruct without this important dimension. The close

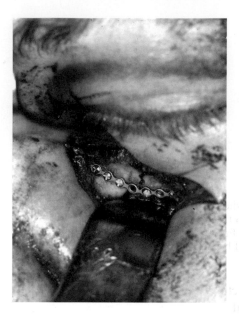

Fig. 14.11   Plating of infraorbital margin fracture.

proximity of the facial nerve to the condylar neck makes the surgical approach taxing and at present the application of IMF for 1–2 weeks is still advocated.

Mid-third fractures

The advent of miniaturised plating systems has allowed the technique of open reduction and internal fixation to be applied to these areas. The same general rules of ORIF apply but as fewer displacing forces are applied to the mid face, smaller plate sizes (1.7–1 mm) can be employed to allow reconstruction of delicate areas such as the infraorbital margins (Fig. 14.11). The concept of reconstruction of the main buttresses of the face is crucial to re-establish the facial geometry. Study models and cast arch bars can be of great value to establish the occlusion pre- and peroperatively and the use of intraoperative IMF is advocated.

Reduction of malar bones and zygomatic arch

The external approach devised by Gillies is made through an incision in the skin above the hairline and over the temporal fossa. It is made at an angle to avoid the terminal branches of the superficial temporal artery. The temporal fascia is exposed and divided to give access to an elevator (Fig. 14.12). This is passed deep to the fascia and to the zygomatic arch. It is used to lift the depressed malar forwards, upwards and outwards (Fig. 14.12). Considerable force is often necessary and the fulcrum must never be the temporal bone, lest the thin lateral wall of the skull be fractured. The assistant keeps the head stabilised while the operator applies the force and checks to

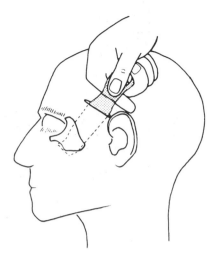

Fig. 14.12   Elevation of left malar showing the incision and a lever in place deep to the malar and zygomatic arch. Note the index finger used as a fulcrum to protect the temporal bone.

ensure that reduction is satisfactory. The malar often clicks into place and is stable without fixation but if not may be held by a bone plate at the zygomatico-frontal suture, the infraorbital margin, or intraorally at the malar buttress. Alternatively an intraosseous pin in the body of the malar may be employed, attached by a vertical bar to a pin placed in the supraorbital rim. The zygoma may also be reduced using a malar hook inserted through a stab incision in line with the lateral canthus at the level of the alar of the nose, although this is not suitable if the zygomatic arch is also depressed. Alternatively an elevator may be passed under the zygoma through a buccal sulcus incision which may be combined with an approach to bone plate fixation at the malar buttress.

In multiple facial injuries the malar should only be fixed after the rest of the maxillary complex has been reduced and immobilised.

Orbital exploration

The orbital floor may require exploration if there is clinical or radiographic evidence of a defect with loss of orbital contents into the maxillary sinus (orbital blowout). Enophthalmos may be masked initially by swelling. Exploration may be combined with reconstruction of the infraorbital margin. Exposure is achieved via infraorbital, blepharoplasty or transconjunctival incisions. Defects may be repaired with bone graft, silastic sheets or titanium mesh. The orbital roof and both walls may also require exploration.

Retrobulbar haemorrhage

This is a severe though rare hazard following reduction of zygomatic fractures or any intervention involving the orbit. Bleeding behind the globe during or after the operation can cause proptosis, pain and decreasing visual acuity which, if the pressure is not relieved, may result in blindness. The blood may be drained

Table 14.4 Retrobulbar haemorrhage.

Signs and symptoms	Time of onset	Treatment	
		Surgical	Medical
Decreasing visual acuity Tunnel vision Eye pain Proptosis	After mid-third trauma, during treatment of zygomatic or Le Fort II/III fractures, after treatment (up to 4 hours)	Drainage of blood from behind eye via infraorbital or lateral canthal incisions	Dexamethasone 20 mg, acetazolamide 1 gm, mannitol 10%, all given IV at onset of symptoms, can be repeated
Eye observations Quarter hourly for 2 hours Half hourly for 2 hours 1 hourly for 2 hours		Observe for Visual acuity Reaction to light Pain	

via an infraorbital or lateral canthal incision; however medical management in the form of steroids, acetazolamide and mannitol can also be successful in reducing the pressure on the optic nerve (Table 14.4). Postoperative eye observations every 15 minutes for 2 hours, then every 30 minutes for 2 hours will aid in the early diagnosis and treatment of this condition.

Le Fort I and II fractures

These can usually be exposed from an intraoral 'horseshoe' incision and the vertical buttress system accurately reduced and fixed at the malar buttress and canine fossa regions. The infraorbital margins may need to be exposed from an extraoral approach and this can allow exploration of the orbital floor if this is involved in the trauma.

Le Fort III fractures

These may require fixation in the same areas depending on the degree of comminution and will require further exposure to allow their fixation to solid bone at the frontozygomatic area and at the nasal bridge. The use of a bicoronal scalp flap gives excellent exposure for the reduction of the fractures in this area. The objective is to rebuild the vertical and horizontal buttress system to re-establish the facial geometry as accurately as possible.

Naso-ethmoidal complex fractures

These fractures, in which the intercanthal distance has been traumatically increased, demand careful diagnosis and management; a bicoronal flap is

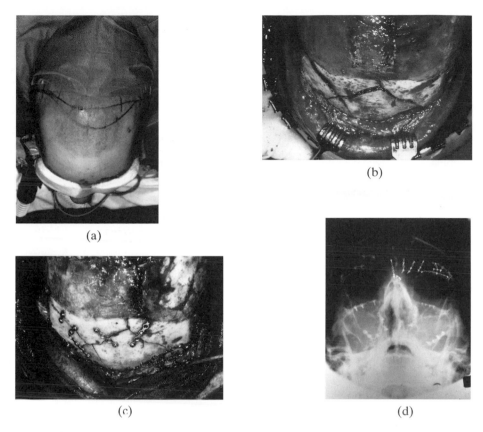

Fig. 14.13 Cranio-facial fractures: (a) bicoronal flap approach; (b) fractures of frontal bone exposed; (c) reconstruction of frontal bone and supraorbital margin; (d) post-operative occipitomental radiograph showing reconstruction of mid-face.

essential to properly reattach the medial canthae and should be undertaken as soon as possible as late repair is extremely difficult (Fig. 14.13).

Edentulous jaws

Though edentulous jaws should be reduced and fixed to obtain satisfactory union, in many cases displacement will be prevented by the periosteum and slight deformity can be compensated for by construction of new dentures. ORIF is still the chosen method of treatment but over-zealous stripping of the periosteum should be avoided as the blood supply to the bone can be severely compromised.

Dentures

The patient's dentures may be used as a guide to the occlusion. These are often immediately available and have the advantage of reproducing both the alveolar ridge and the patient's bite accurately.

Table 14.5   Surgical approaches to the facial bones.

	Intraoral		Extraoral	
	Area	Approach	Area	Approach
mandible	Angle Body Parasymphysis Symphysis	Incision below attached gingivae	Condyle Lower border	Retro-mandibular, preauricular Sub-mandibular
zygoma	Malar buttress	Incision below attached gingivae	Zygomatico- frontal suture Infraorbital margin Zygomatic arch	Brow Blepharoplasty Infraorbital Preauricular bicoronal
maxilla	Malar buttress Canine fossa	Incision below attached gingivae extending to 'horseshoe'	As for zygoma + supraorbital	As above Bicoronal
naso-ethmoidal			Nasal bridge Medial canthae	Bicoronal

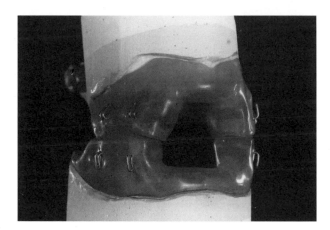

Fig. 14.14   Gunnings splints for use in an edentulous mandible.

Gunning's splints

These are the standard splint for immobilising edentulous jaws. They are an upper and lower bite block made in acrylic. They have a shallow periphery, a hole anteriorly for feeding, and cleats for intermaxillary fixation. They are constructed from casts of the patient's dentures, which are also used to register the bite, or by direct impressions of the patient's jaws when the bite is registered using conventional bite blocks (Fig. 14.14).

Where there is displacement neither a satisfactory impression nor bite recording is possible, and the fitting surface of the splint is lined with gutta percha and moulded to the jaw *after* the fragments have been reduced. By placing gutta percha in previously prepared gutters on the occlusal surface, the bite can also be corrected.

Gunning's splints or dentures may be wired to the jaws to reduce the bone fragments, following which IMF may be applied.

Circumferential and transalveolar wiring

In the lower jaw three wires are used, one on each side in the first molar region and one anteriorly. The wire is put in place by passing a curved Kelsey Fry awl (Fig. 14.15) through an extraoral stab incision up into the mouth on the lingual side and then pulling a wire under the jaw to the buccal side, keeping the point as close to bone as possible to avoid the lingual and facial arteries. The upper splint may be attached to underlying bone with titanium mini-plate screws or held in position by transalveolar wires, one on each side in the molar region and one anteriorly (Fig. 14.15).

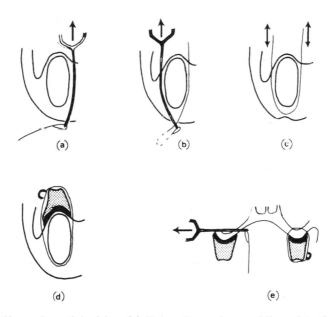

Fig. 14.15   Circumferential wiring. (a) Kelsey Fry awl passed lingual to the mandible. (b) Wire alongside lingual side of mandible and the awl passed bucally to pick up extraoral end of the wire. (c) Sawing through soft tissue to ensure close apposition of wire on bone. (d) Lower splint lined with gutta percha wired in place. (e) *Left*, straight awl passed through maxillary alveolus and across the antral floor to draw transalveolar wire through from palate. *Right*, transalveolar wire in place to hold upper Gunning's splint.

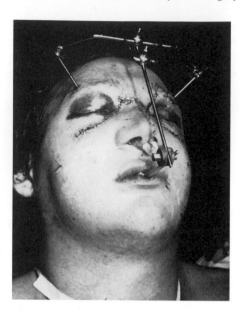

Fig. 14.16   Levant frame attached to upper metal cap splint by bars and universal joints. Note facial laceration extended for open reduction.

The following methods are used infrequently in maxillary fractures in patients who will not tolerate the extended surgical time required for ORIF.

Craniomaxillary fixation

The maxilla may be fixed to the skull to hold it firmly in place. This is done by attaching metal rods to locking plates on arch bars or Gunnings splints. These rods come out of the mouth and are connected by means of universal joints (Clouston-Walker joints) and rods to a metal halo frame or supraorbital intraosseous pins joined by a connecting bar (Levant frame) (Fig. 14.16).

Halo head frame

This is screwed to the head by means of pins which penetrate the skin and engage the outer bony cortical plate of the skull. Two pairs of opposing pins in the occipital and frontal regions are placed above the hairline to avoid unsightly scars. The temporal vessels should be identified to avoid damage to these when placing the frontal pins. Once in position rods from arch bars will provide rigid fixation of the maxilla.

Supraorbital pins and frame

Pins are placed via an eyebrow incision. Holes are drilled into the supraorbital bone using a brace and bit and a self-tapping pin is inserted to engage both cortical plates without penetrating the inner. The pins are then joined using a Levant frame and this is connected to the teeth via rods (Fig. 14.16).

Internal suspension

In Le Fort I fractures 0.5 mm stainless steel wire is passed round the zygomatic arches using an awl inserted via a skin incision through the mucosa beneath the arch in the upper buccal sulcus. A wire is threaded through the hole in the awl and drawn upwards over the zygomatic arch and back down on the lateral side into the mouth. This wire is attached either to cleats on arch bars or eyelet wires.

Complications of fractures

Removal of bone plates

Infrequently titanium bone plates will have to be removed. This is due to patient request, plate exposure or, rarely, involvement of the plate in infection. The most frequent area from which plates are removed in the mandible is the parasymphyseal region and in the maxilla at the zygomatico-frontal suture region. The plates should ideally remain until bone healing is complete before removal, unless rigid fixation is lost due to loosening of the screws or breakage of the plate.

Delayed union

Normally fractures unite in about 4–8 weeks, but take longer in elderly patients. This time may be greatly increased in comminuted, compound or infected fractures. Rigid internal fixation will allow these fractures to heal but some may take several months during which time they must be carefully observed. Radiographs may be taken at intervals if movement of the fracture is evident clinically, to determine whether non-union has occurred (Fig. 14.17).

Malunion

This is union with the bone ends still misplaced or badly reduced. It may be slight and cause the patient little disability or it may be such as to interfere with function or appearance. Slight deformity affecting the occlusion can be treated by grinding or extracting teeth, and the provision of dentures. More severe deformities may require re-fracture, and reapposition of the bone ends by an osteotomy operation.

Non-union

This term refers to the failure to obtain bony union, where healing has occurred by fibrous union only. In facial trauma it is significant only in the mandible. Clinically movement is found across the fracture line. On radiographs a smoothing over of the bone ends is seen, which is later followed by a deposition of cortical bone (eburnation). The chief causes of non-union are a failure to achieve satisfactory apposition, bone loss and movement or infection in the fracture line. Treatment of non-union is necessary in the body of the mandible but may be acceptable in the ascending ramus and the condyle, if function is unimpaired.

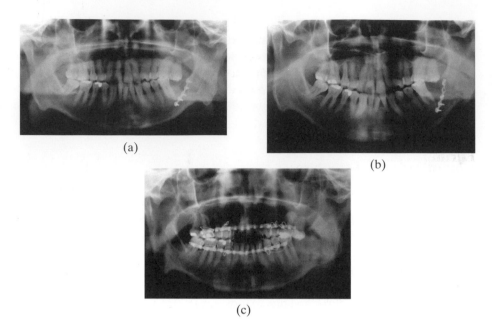

(a)

(b)

(c)

Fig. 14.17   Loss of fixation: (a) good reduction of fracture at left angle (b) three weeks post-operatively – note loss of screws and movement of fracture (c) IMF applied with arch bars following removal of fixation. The patient may have been involved in further trauma.

Bone loss

In severe injuries, particularly in gunshot wounds, there may be bone loss. In the mandible, if this is slight, a satisfactory result can be achieved by approximating the bone ends. Otherwise, the gap is accepted and the fragments are reduced into their normal position and held there by splints, long bone plates or external pin fixation. When soft tissue healing has taken place and the inflammatory reaction has settled, the defect is repaired with bone grafts. This may be delayed several weeks, or even months.

Infection

This may reach the fracture from wounds in the skin or more commonly from the mouth. The mandible is more susceptible to infection than the maxilla. In the latter, drainage is downward into the mouth and the thin plates of bone with a good blood supply make it more resistant to infection. Infection from the mouth may enter the fracture through a tear in the mucous membrane, from dead teeth, particularly those in the line of fracture, or by direct or lymphatic spread from other infected teeth in the jaw. If rigid fixation has been achieved with a bio-inert material, such as titanium, fracture healing should continue if energetic treatment with antibacterial drugs and drainage, together with the removal of infected teeth, is instituted. On rare occasions the fixation may have to be removed and IMF applied.

Residual trismus

In mandibular fractures residual trismus may be due to scarring in the traumatised muscles or rarely due to ankylosis in intracapsular condylar fractures. In poorly reduced zygomatic arch fractures bony interference may occur with the coronoid process. The cause must be carefully ascertained and treated either surgically or with exercises and physiotherapy.

Further reading

Champy, M., Lodde, J.P., Jaegar, J.H., Wilk, A. & Gerber, J.C. (1978) Mandibular osteosynthesis by miniature screwed plates via a buccal approach. *J. Maxillofac. Surg.*, **6**, 14.

Hawkesford, J. & Banks, J.G. (1994) *Maxillofacial and Dental Emergencies.* Oxford University Press, Oxford.

Williams, J.L. (ed.) (1994) *Rowe and Williams Maxillofacial Injuries.* Churchill Livingstone, Edinburgh.

Advanced Trauma Life Support Student Manual (1997) American College of Surgeons. Chicago, Illinois.

Symposium on management of the bilateral fractured condyle (1998) *J. Oral Surgery*, **27**, 244–67.

Chapter 15
Tumours of the Mouth and the Management of Oral Cancer

- Oral precancer
- Oral cancer
- Aetiology and risk factors
- Clinical presentation
- Spread of oral cancer
- Principles of management
- Surgery
- Radiotherapy
- Chemotherapy
- Recent advances

A tumour is a swelling or mass caused by excessive, continued growth of cells within a tissue; growth is unco-ordinated with that of normal tissue and persists in the same excessive manner after cessation of the stimulus that evoked it, in distinction to developmental abnormalities such as haemangiomas which are termed hamartomas. Tumours may be either benign or malignant (Table 15.1).

Oncology is the study and science of new growths, while a neoplasm refers to any new, diseased form of tissue growth. Cancer is the overall name applied to malignant growths, over 90% of which are derived from epithelial tissues, and is essentially a genetic disease, caused by somatic mutation. The multi-stage theory of carcinogenesis believes that individual cancers arise from several sequential mutations in cellular DNA. There is a close correlation between cancer incidence and increased age, reflecting the time required to accumulate the critical number of genetic abnormalities needed for malignant change.

The two most significant characteristics of malignant growths are: local invasion, in which malignant cells either singularly or as cords or sheets infiltrate and destroy adjacent normal tissue, and metastasis in which secondary tumours, by dissemination of tumour emboli through lymphatic and vascular channels, are formed at sites discontinuous from the primary. Death from cancer usually results from tumour deposition within vital organs such as the liver, lungs or brain, from a generalised carcinomatosis, or from uncontrolled disease at the primary site causing airway obstruction or haemorrhage from large blood vessels.

Table 15.1 Benign tumours of the mouth.

Pathological characteristics	Clinical features	Common oral tumours	Treatment
Slow growing Expansile Localised Encapsulated Well differentiated	Mucosal or submucosal swelling Local pressure or displacement effects	Squamous cell papilloma Adenoma Fibroma Neuro-fibroma Lipoma Osteoma	Local excision

Table 15.2 Oral precancer.

Classification	Definition (WHO 1978)	Clinical examples
Precancerous lesions	Morphologically altered tissue in which cancer is more likely to occur than in its apparently normal counterpart	Leukoplakia Erythroplakia Speckled leukoplakia
Precancerous Conditions	Generalised states associated with a significantly increased risk of cancer	Immunosuppression Submucous fibrosis Sideropaenic dysphagia Discoid lupus erythematosus Actinic keratosis Lichen planus Syphilis

Oral precancer

Fundamental to reducing cancer morbidity and mortality is the ability to recognise the earliest possible neoplastic changes in oral tissues. Dental practitioners have a unique opportunity during routine oral examination to detect malignant neoplasms while they are asymptomatic and often precancerous. In 1978 the World Health Organisation (WHO) divided oral precancer into: precancerous lesions, altered tissues in which oral cancer is more likely to occur, and precancerous conditions, which are generalised states associated with a significantly increased risk of cancer (Table 15.2).

Epithelial dysplasia is defined as a collection of epithelial changes seen by light microscopy (primarily disordered tissue maturation and disturbed cellular proliferation) and is the most important determinant of the risk of malignant transformation of precancerous lesions. Pathologists qualitatively divide dysplasia into mild, moderate, severe or carcinoma-in-situ depending on the extent of dysplastic features and the resultant risk of malignant change.

Table 15.3   Management protocol for oral precancer.

(1) Eliminate risk factors – tobacco, alcohol
(2) Clinical photographic record
(3) Baseline haematology – full blood count, serum ferritin, B_{12}, folate
(4) Candidal swab
(5) Incisional biopsy and dysplasia characterisation
(6) Careful clinical follow-up and consider repeat biopsy for mild dysplasias
(7) Laser excision for moderate/severe dysplasias
(8) Long-term clinical follow up
(9) Monitor oral mucosa for field change

Epithelial dysplasia does not mean that a lesion will inevitably proceed to an invasive cancer, but an increased risk exists which worsens as the epithelium becomes increasingly dysplastic. Erythroplakic lesions generally contain more severely dysplastic epithelium than leukoplakia, and carry a higher risk of malignant change, as do speckled (red and white) lesions, whilst rough or nodular leukoplakias carry more risk than smooth (homogeneous) leukoplakias. Lesions arising in the floor of mouth and ventral tongue display higher rates of malignant transformation than other oral sites.

Table 15.3 outlines a pragmatic management protocol for patients with oral precancer. Laser surgery, a technique involving high temperature tissue vaporisation and coagulative necrosis, allows accurate dissection and excision of premalignant lesions with reduced morbidity; minimal blood loss, reduction in post-operative pain, reduced scarring and rapid healing without skin grafting facilitate an acceptable strategy in patients for whom multiple or recurrent oral lesions are not uncommon.

Field change

An important complicating factor is that following surgical removal of individual precancerous lesions the rest of the patient's upper aerodigestive tract mucosa may display widespread precancerous change, rendering patients susceptible to other primary cancers of larynx, oesophagus and lungs.

Oral cancer

Whilst the term oral cancer encompasses a range of malignant tumours arising within the lip, oral cavity and oropharynx (Table 15.4), over 90% of oral cancers are primary squamous cell carcinomas arising from the oral mucous membrane.

Worldwide, the incidence of oral cancer varies, with India and parts of Asia having the highest rates (40% of all cancers), while in western countries the incidence is about 3% of all new cancers. However this incidence is rising, particularly in younger patients and women, and oral cancer is a particularly lethal

Table 15.4   Malignancies of the oral cavity.

Primary tumours	Squamous cell carcinoma (>90%) Minor salivary gland carcinomas Lymphoma Malignant melanoma Sarcoma
Secondary tumours (Metastases)	Adenocarcinomas primarily from breast, renal and gastrointestinal tract primaries

disease. Approximately 3400 new cases of oral cancer occur each year in the UK and there are about 1600 deaths.

Overall the 5 year survival rate for patients with oral cancer is only 50%, although small, slow-growing lesions, tumours detected early and those presenting at the front of the mouth tend to do better. Posteriorly sited, rapidly growing tumours invading bone and with demonstrable lymph node metastases at presentation have the worst prognosis.

Aetiology and risk factors

The principal aetiological factors involve the use of tobacco and alcohol, which are known mucosal irritants and mutagenic agents. There is an important synergistic relationship between the two, which significantly increases the risk of cancer for those who both smoke and drink.

Patients who have had oral cancer previously, or those who have had lung, throat or oesophageal tumours, are also at high risk of developing new oral tumours or recurrence of their original cancers. Immunocompromised patients, such as those with AIDS or post-transplant patients on long term immunosuppressive agents, are also at risk. Other postulated aetiological agents include viruses, chronic candidal infections, anaemias, nutritional and vitamin deficiencies, and for lip cancer exposure to ultra-violet radiation.

Clinical presentation

The most frequent clinical presentation is an indurated area of ulceration, often surrounded by leukoplakic or erythroplakic patches, while the commonest sites involved are the floor of the mouth, ventro-lateral tongue and the soft palate complex (soft palate, retromolar trigone and anterior tonsillar pillar).

Oral cancer is usually asymptomatic in the early stages. Late presentation is common although patients report non-specific symptoms over several months prior to their seeking attention. (Table 15.5 summarises the salient signs and symptoms suspicious of oral malignancy.)

Table 15.5 Clinical presentation of oral cancers.

Symptoms	Early lesions	Asymptomatic
		Irritation
		Discomfort
	Late lesions	Pain and swelling
		Paraesthesia
		Dysarthia
		Dysphagia
Signs	Non-healing ulcer	
	Induration and fixation of tissues	
	Exophytic growth	
	White/red mucosal patches	
	Unexplained localised tooth mobility	
	Non-healing tooth socket	

Table 15.6 Spread of oral cancer.

(1) Local invasion	Soft tissues and muscles
	Perineural spaces
	Blood vessels
	Bone
(2) Regional lymph node metastasis	
(3) Distant spread	Lungs
	Liver
	Bones

Spread of oral cancer

The most significant behavioural feature of oral cancers is their ability to invade and destroy local structures and to spread via lymphatics into the neck (Table 15.6). An appreciation of the pattern of spread is essential for effective treatment in order to control the disease within the mouth and neck.

Local invasion

Cancers can infiltrate widely into adjacent connective tissue, within muscle bundles, perineural spaces or local blood vessels. Direct extension via periodontal membrane or cortical deficiencies in edentulous ridges allows invasion of alveolar bone.

Lymph node metastasis

The likelihood of lymphatic spread increases with the size of the primary tumour. While the precise group of cervical lymph nodes affected depends on the location of the primary, intraoral cancers tend to spread initially to ipsilateral submandibular, upper, middle and lower deep cervical nodes (Levels

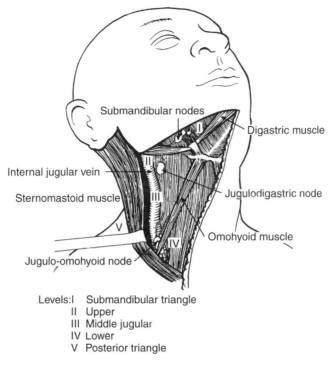

Levels: I Submandibular triangle
     II Upper
     III Middle jugular
     IV Lower
     V Posterior triangle

Fig. 15.1 Surgical anatomy of cervical lymph node groups. Levels: I submandibular triangle; II upper; III middle jugular; IV lower; V posterior triangle.

I to IV in Figure 15.1). Tumours of the tongue, lip and floor of mouth close to the midline can metastasise to nodes on both sides of the neck, while the posterior triangle (Level V in Fig. 15.1) may be involved in aggressive tongue and posterior oral tumours. The more lymph nodes involved, the presence of metastases in lower cervical nodes and the extension of tumour beyond the node capsule (extra-capsular spread) all herald a worse prognosis.

Distant spread

Distant spread tends to be more frequent in the later stages of the disease and may not be clinically apparent, although metastatic deposits have been found in the lungs, liver and bones in approximately 50% of post-mortem examinations carried out in patients dying with oral cancer.

Principles of management

The management of patients with oral cancer presents considerable challenges and it is mandatory that an experienced and specialised multidisciplinary head and neck oncology team are involved in all stages of assessment, treatment and

Table 15.7   Multidisciplinary head and neck oncology team.

Medical and dental staff
- Consultant head and neck surgeons (from maxillofacial, ENT and plastic surgery specialities)
- Consultant clinical oncologist (radiotherapy and chemotherapy expertise)
- Consultant in restorative dentistry
- Consultant in oral/head and neck pathology
- Access to consultants in radiology and diagnostic imaging
- Access to specialists in palliative medicine

Specialist nursing services
- Clinical nurse specialisation in head and neck surgery
- Macmillan palliative care specialists

Paramedical support services
- Speech therapists
- Dieticians
- Physiotherapists
- Maxillofacial laboratory and prosthetic services
- Access to psychological care services

Table 15.8   Principles of oral cancer management.

(1) Thorough evaluation of the patient and their disease
(2) Tumour diagnosis, classification and disease staging
(3) Comprehensive treatment planning
(4) Co-ordination of therapeutic modalities (e.g. combination of surgery and radiotherapy)
(5) Post-treatment oral reconstruction and rehabilitation
(6) Psychological and social support

follow up (Table 15.7). The overall aim of treatment is to eliminate the primary tumour and any neck node metastases, while minimising patient morbidity. The basic principles applied to the clinical management of oral cancer are listed in Table 15.8.

Evaluation of disease

Accurate assessment of the extent of disease is important and includes a detailed clinical history, general medical review and physical examination, a biopsy of the primary tumour to confirm the diagnosis and histology, possibly an examination under anaesthesia (EUA) to facilitate inspection, palpation and measurement of larger, painful and posteriorly sited lesions, and an evaluation of cervical lymph node involvement. Endoscopic examination of the rest of the upper aerodigestive tract may be carried out to identify other primary (syn-

Table 15.9   Investigations used in oral cancer assessment.

Classification	Types	Specific aims
Histopathological examination	Incisional tissue biopsy	To confirm clinical diagnosis Classify tumour differentiation
	Fine needle aspiration (FNA) cytology	To confirm presence of metastatic carcinoma in enlarged lymph nodes
Diagnostic imaging	Plain radiography	
	• Orthopantomogram	To establish jaw bone or tooth involvement
	• Occipitomental view	To assess maxillary sinus or orbital involvement
	• Chest X-ray	Screening for bronchial cancer or metastatic lung disease
	CT scanning	Particularly useful in imaging bony involvement and antral and pterygoid regions
	MR scanning	Ideally suited for soft tissue tumours and cervical node assessment
Laboratory investigations	Haematology	To identify underlying anaemias or clotting disorders
	Blood chemistry	To identify renal or liver disease (e.g. cirrhosis, metastases)

chronous) tumours. Table 15.9 details the important further investigations carried out during the assessment phase.

Classification and staging

Evaluation allows classification of cancers according to the size of the primary tumour (T), the involvement of associated regional lymph nodes (N) and the presence of distant metastases (M). Using the TNM system, it is then possible to stage individual patients' disease. This allows meaningful treatment planning and assessment of prognosis and helps advise patients and relatives, as well as providing a meaningful reference for data analysis between different treatment centres (Table 15.10).

Treatment planning

The fundamental decision of whether curative or palliative treatment is appropriate follows discussion within the multidisciplinary team and between patients and their relatives. While the aim of curative treatment is clearly the

Table 15.10   Classification and staging of oral cancers.

TNM Classification:	Clinical assessment of the anatomical extent of disease
Tumour	$T_1 < 2$ cm
	$T_2 < 2$–4 cm
	$T_3 > 4$ cm
	T_4 Infiltrating deep structures
Nodes	N_1 Mobile palpable nodes <3 cm on same side
	N_2 Contra or bilateral mobile nodes 3–6 cm
	N_3 Fixed node(s) >6 cm
Metastases	M_1 Distant metastases present
Resultant Clinical Staging:	Standard communicable description of individual patients' disease
Stage I	$\mathbf{T_1}$ No Mo
Stage II	$\mathbf{T_2}$ No Mo
Stage III	$\mathbf{T_3}$ No Mo
	or
	$T_1/T_2/T_3$ $\mathbf{N_1}$ Mo
Stage IV	$\mathbf{T_4}$
	Any T $\mathbf{N_2/N_3}$ Mo
	Any T/Any N/$\mathbf{M_1}$

elimination of disease with minimum morbidity, palliative care aims to improve and prolong the symptom-free phase of the patient's life with the recognition that the disease is unlikely to be completely eradicated.

The choice is then whether to use surgery or radiotherapy as the primary treatment. If surgery is chosen, radiotherapy may be used in an adjuvant manner post-operatively. If radiotherapy is used as primary treatment, surgery is reserved for salvage therapy to deal with any residual disease. However, following radiotherapy tissues have a reduced blood supply and exhibit marked fibrosis leading to delayed healing and the risk of wound breakdown and fistula formation. The general health, age, life expectancy and wishes of the patient must be taken into consideration during treatment planning. While surgery may necessitate the loss of important functional units such as the lips, tongue or mandible, radiotherapy may produce immediate morbidity (stomatitis and xerostomia) or longer term problems such as osteoradionecrosis.

Surgery

Surgical access

Good surgical access is fundamental to the effective exposure and complete removal of oral tumours. The approach adopted should be easy to repair and produce minimal scarring and deformity. While an intraoral technique may be sufficient for small anteriorly sited tumours, splitting of the lip, division of the mandible (mandibulotomy) and resultant mandibular swing fully displays the posterior tongue, retromolar and soft palate regions and facilitates tumour excision in three dimensions under direct vision. Facial cheek flaps and maxillary osteotomies allow similar access to the posterior palate and retromaxillary regions.

Resection of the primary tumour

The principal objective of surgical treatment is to excise the entire primary tumour with a margin (ideally about 1 cm) of adjacent normal tissue in anticipation of microscopic spread, and to remove potential channels of metastasis such as nerves, vessels and lymphatics.

Lower lip cancers may be treated by wedge excision alone or combined with a lip shave procedure (removal of the entire vermilion) where there is extensive ultra-violet damage. Anterior tongue tumours may require partial, hemi or subtotal glossectomy depending on the size and position. While small buccal mucosal cancers can be excised intraorally, more advanced lesions may require excision of buccinator muscle and overlying skin.

Tumours of the floor of mouth, retromolar region and lower alveolus usually involve the underlying mandible and require mandibular resection. As bony invasion usually occurs from the superior aspect, a marginal resection may be possible preserving the mandibular lower border. The inferior dental nerve canal, extending from lingula to mental foramen, should be included in mandibular body resections owing to the likelihood of perineural spread.

Mucosal excision, alveolar resection, palatal fenestration or maxillectomy may be required for tumours arising from the palatal mucosa and maxillary alveolus depending on their size and position.

Management of the neck

Dissection of cervical lymph nodes containing metastatic disease is essential for the effective management of oral cancer, and is indicated whenever clinical examination or imaging techniques confirm enlarged, draining lymph nodes. FNA may be carried out to confirm cytologically the presence of carcinoma deposits within enlarged nodes.

Neck dissection operations may be classified according to the various levels at which nodes are removed and the key anatomical structures which are either excised or preserved (Table 15.11). In oral cancer management, Levels I to III or IV are the most often dissected, with post-operative radiotherapy advised if multiple nodes prove positive or there is extracapsular tumour spread.

Neck dissection may be contraindicated, however, in extensive disease where involved lymph nodes may be fixed by tumour extension into vital structures such as the carotid artery or skull base. A complete surgical excision is either not possible or may produce significant morbidity or even mortality.

Table 15.11   Neck dissection operations.

Comprehensive (Nodes excised from levels I to V)	(a) Radical (no structures preserved) (b) Modified radical (preservation of sternomastoid muscle, internal jugular vein and accessory nerve)
Selective	e.g. Supra omohyoid (nodes excised from levels I to III/IV only)

Table 15.12   Reconstructive techniques.

(1) Primary closure (soft tissue defects)
(2) 'Simple' free grafts
    Skin   Split thickness
                Full thickness
    Bone   Cortical
                Cancellous
(3) Local flap repair
    Intraoral tissue   tongue flap
                        Buccal fat pad
    Facial skin   e.g. nasolabial flap
    Muscle   e.g. temporalis flap
(4) Regional pedicled flaps e.g. pectoralis major muscle and skin flap
(5) Free flaps (microvascular tissue transfer)
    Radial forearm flap
    Fibula flap
    Groin and iliac crest flap
(6) Alloplastic techniques
    Titanium reconstruction plates, mesh trays and implants
    Acrylic dentofacial prostheses and obturators

Reconstruction

Following ablative tumour surgery, reconstruction is essential to prevent facial deformity, maintain bone continuity and facilitate masticatory, swallowing and speech functions. Reduction of psychological morbidity and an acceptable quality of life outcome are equally important aims. Extensive removal of orofacial soft tissues and underlying mandibular or maxillary bone is often necessary for effective tumour resection and a range of reconstructive techniques are available (Table 15.12).

The use of free tissue transfer and microvascular surgery, in which free flaps (often comprising skin, muscle and bone) are transferred from distant sites and their dependent arteries and veins connected to vessels in the neck, enables reconstruction of complex defects with vascularised tissue at the time of tumour excision. The radial forearm osseofasciocutaneous flap, a groin flap based on the deep circumflex iliac artery (DCIA), or the fibula flap, may be used to reconstruct the mandible (Fig. 15.2).

Maxillary defects result in direct communications between oral and nasal cavities or the paranasal sinuses, with the inevitable production of nasal speech

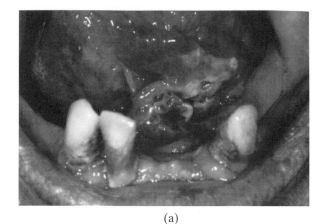

Fig. 15.2   Stages in the surgical management of a floor of mouth cancer: (a) Typical clinical appearance of an exophytic and infiltrative floor of mouth squamous cell carcinoma.

(a)

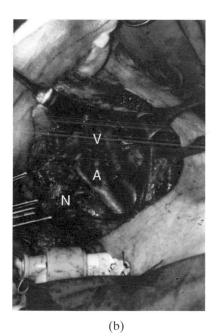

(b)

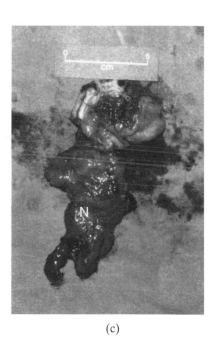

(c)

Fig. 15.2   (b) Functional neck dissection in progress demonstrating the internal jugular vein (V) and the common carotid arterial system (A). The sternomastoid muscle is retracted posteriorly and the fatty tissue containing the lymph nodes is being dissected anteriorly (N).

Fig. 15.2   (c) 'In continuity' resection specimen includes the mandibular gingiva, floor of mouth and anterior tongue, together with the draining cervical lymph nodes (N).

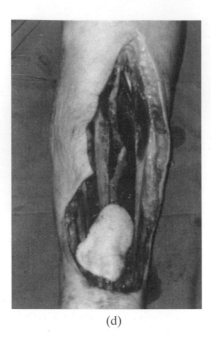

(d)

Fig. 15.2   (d) Free fascio-cutaneous forearm flap and vascular pedicle (radial artery plus venae comitantes) being raised.

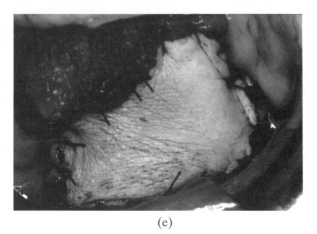

(e)

Fig. 15.2   (e) Forearm flap transferred to oral defect and secured in place with multiple interrupted sutures.

and swallowing difficulties. The principal aim is thus to re-establish palatal continuity either with flap reconstruction or a prosthetic appliance and obturator which fills the defect. Initially, such appliances may be secured with intraosseous screws to adjacent palatal bone holding skin grafts in position to reline mucosal defects. Later, they are replaced with specially designed removable appliances.

Table 15.13   The role of radiotherapy in oral cancer treatment.

Indications for radiotherapy	Patient unfit for major surgery Tumour inaccessible or technically unresectable by surgery Surgery likely to produce severe deformity or functional morbidity Patient unwilling to undergo surgery
Contraindications to radiotherapy	Previous local irradiation Large tumours, with bony invasion and cervical lymph node metastases Unreliable patient attendance for out-patient therapy

Radiotherapy

Radiotherapy is the treatment of tumours with ionising radiation and is potentially curative in oral cancer treatment (Table 15.13). X-ray, gamma ray and less commonly particulate radiation is delivered as external beams from outside the patient (teletherapy) or radioactive materials such as iridium wires can be implanted within or in close proximity to the tumour (brachytherapy).

External beams of supervoltage radiation converge on the tumour, so the latter receives a very much high dose than the surrounding tissues. The total therapeutic dose of external beam therapy, usually 60 Grays (Gy), is fractionated into a number of smaller doses over 4 to 6 weeks. This increases the differential effect on tumour cells which are less able to repair themselves compared with normal tissue. Brachytherapy treatment requires an intense radiation dose within the tumour and immediate vicinity, usually delivering a total of 65 to 70 Gy over 8 days.

Radiation may be given palliatively to incurable patients with a short life expectancy to relieve disease symptoms such as pain, bleeding or swelling. A cure is not attempted and the risk of acute reaction lessened by using a smaller dose, for example, 20 Gy over 5 days.

Biological effects of radiation

Intracellular free radicals are formed leading to DNA damage and ultimately cell death when mitosis is attempted. Mitotic death occurs within a few days in rapidly proliferating tumours such as squamous cell carcinoma. The effectiveness of radiotherapy is increased in radiosensitive tumours, in the presence of increased oxygenation and in smaller tumours. In a successful treatment the tumour regresses and is replaced by scar tissue. Mitotic death of normal cells produces the side effects of radiotherapy.

Rapidly proliferating tissues such as oral mucosa and skin affected after 14 to 21 days (acute reactions) lead to mucositis, loss of taste, and erythema and alopecia respectively. These acute effects usually heal completely as the normal tissues proliferate and recover. Late reactions, which are irreversible, occur due to devascularisation of irradiated tissues as a result of mitotic death of slowly replicating vascular endothelial cells.

Xerostomia

Irradiation of salivary gland tissue produces an acute permanent loss of secretory cells. Salivary flow reduces during the first few days of radiotherapy, but within 6 weeks has stopped completely. The resulting dryness of the mouth can be distressing to patients, adds to their oral discomfort and impairs taste, chewing and swallowing.

Xerostomia carries an increased risk of rapidly destructive dental caries (radiation caries) and advanced periodontal disease. Artificial saliva preparations may be helpful, while oral administration of pilocarpine may help increase flow in patients with some residual salivary gland function.

Osteoradionecrosis

Bone irradiation lethally damages both osteoblasts and osteoclasts so that when stimulated to divide, as a result of a traumatic stimulus such as a dental extraction or localised infection, mitotic death occurs precipitating necrosis. There is also diminished vascularity of the periosteum due to late effects on endothelial lining cells, particularly involving the dense and less vascular mandibular bone.

Clinically, the radionecrotic process usually starts as an ulceration on the alveolar mucosa with brownish dead bone exposed at the base. Pathological fracture may occur in the weakened bone, but the process may not be painful until secondary infection ensues when severe discomfort, trismus, foetor oris and general malaise predominate. Radiographically, the earliest changes are a 'moth-eaten' appearance of the bone, followed by sequestration.

Treatment is predominantly conservative with long-term antibiotic therapy and careful removal of sequestra when necessary. In intractable cases, extensive surgical resection and reconstruction with compound muscle and bone flaps may be necessary. Hyperbaric oxygen and ultrasound therapy have also been recommended.

Dental care for oncology patients

Assessment of the general dental state by a specialist in restorative dentistry is mandatory for all head and neck cancer patients, especially for those likely to undergo radiotherapy. Extractions are advised for carious, non-vital, periodontally involved teeth or retained roots and their removal is performed carefully pre-radiotherapy to ensure rapid healing.

Subsequent to radiotherapy, meticulous oral hygiene is essential especially during treatment when the mouth is inflamed and sore. Dilute chlorhexidine mouthwashes, topical fluoride applications, saliva substitutes and active restorative care may all be needed to preserve the remaining dentition. Should a tooth have to be extracted it is essential that an atraumatic surgical technique is used, together with antibiotic cover until healing is complete.

Chemotherapy

Chemotherapy has provided a major advance in the management of certain malignancies. As the primary form of treatment for lymphomas and leukaemias, for example, chemotherapeutic agents have markedly improved the long-term survival rates of patients. In general, however, chemotherapy is less effective in treating solid tumours in adults and is rarely of curative value in oral cancer treatment, but may have a role in trying to prevent secondary tumours developing from metastatic deposits.

Chemotherapy targets actively dividing cells to eliminate tumours while allowing normal cells to recover and repair. Drugs are thus usually administered in high doses intermittently and often in combination to aid synergy and overcome potential resistance. Many types of drugs are now available (Table 15.14), and a number of different therapeutic regimes may be applied (Table 15.15).

The major side effects of chemotherapy are nausea and vomiting, bone marrow suppression, alopecia and oral mucositis. To reduce the severity of mucositis, a high standard of oral hygiene and careful attention to preventive and restorative dental care is essential.

Recent advances and current problems in oral cancer management

Unfortunately, overall survival rates for oral cancer have changed little over the last 20 years, although accurate disease staging and effective treatment planning (combination therapy involving both surgery and radiotherapy) have produced more effective loco-regional disease control. Greater number of patients now

Table 15.14   Chemotherapeutic drugs.

Classification	Mode of action	Drugs used in oral cancer treatment
Alkylating agents	Form cross-links between DNA strands	CIS-platinum Bleomycin
Antimetabolites	Impair synthesis and assembly of purine and pyrimidine DNA bases	Methotrexate 5-fluoruracil
Mitotic inhibitors	Disrupt microtubules essential for cell division	Vincristine

Table 15.15   Chemotherapy treatment regimes.

Type	Administration	Aim
Induction	Prior to surgery or radiotherapy	To reduce tumour size and kill tumour cells
Sandwich	Between surgery and radiotherapy	To reduce risk of metastases
Adjuvant	After surgery or radiotherapy	To improve disease-free survival
Concurrent	In conjunction with radiotherapy	To sensitise tumour cells and increase destructive effects of radiotherapy
Palliative	After all other treatments	Shrink persistent tumour masses. Pain relief

die, however, from distant metastases or from the emergence of second or even third primary tumours.

Future developments in oral cancer therapy will require effective public health measures to target high risk population groups and wider introduction of active preventive therapies. Accurate, reproducible and predictive clinico-pathological assessments of individual precancer and cancerous lesions are required, and further research is both necessary and ongoing into the potential therapeutic role of newer genetic and immunological therapies.

Further reading

Brown, A.E. & Langdon, J.D. (1995) Management of oral cancer. *Ann. R. Coll. Surg. Engl.*, **77**, 404–408.

Cawson, R.A., Langdon, J.D. & Eveson, J.W. (1996) *Surgical Pathology of the Mouth and Jaws*. Wright, Oxford.

Dimitroulis, G. & Avery, B.S. (1998) *Oral Cancer: A Synopsis of Pathology and Management*. Butterworth Heinemann, Oxford.

Langdon, J.D. & Henk, J.M. (1995) *Malignant Tumours of the Mouth, Jaws and Salivary Glands*. Edward Arnold, London.

Silverman, S. (1998) *Oral Cancer*, 4th edn, American Cancer Society. B.C. Decker Inc, Hamilton, Canada.

Speight, P.M. & Morgan, P.R. (1993) The Natural History and Pathology of Oral Cancer and Precancer. *Community Dental Health* **10**(Suppl. 1), 31–41.

Chapter 16
Treatment of Surgical Conditions of the Salivary Glands

- Presenting complaints
- Minor salivary glands
- Major salivary glands
- Specific conditions

The diseases of the salivary glands that may be treated by surgery include cysts, salivary calculi, infections and tumours.

Presenting complaints

Presenting complaints may include the appearance of a mass whose size and growth rate should be recorded, together with how long it has been present and the presence/absence of symptoms. In addition any change in consistency of the saliva or taste sensation should be noted. Ascertain if there is involvement of other systems such as the eyes, liver, lungs or joints. Where a swelling is present

Table 16.1 Classification of salivary gland disorders.

Congenital	Aplasia
	Hypoplasia
Inflammatory	Sialadenitis – viral or bacterial infection
	Auto-immune – Sjörgen's
	Idiopathic – necrotising sialometaplasia
	Sarcoidosis
Traumatic	Mucocele, ranula
	Salivary fistulae
	Post-irradiation sialadenitis
Obstructive	Sialolithiasis
	Atrasia or ductal stenosis
Tumours	Benign – pleomorphic adenoma
	Malignant – mucoepidermoid carcinoma, acinic cell carcinoma, adenocarcinoma, adenoid cystic carcinoma
Idiopathic	Sialosis

it should be noted whether this is intermittent, with persistent pain related to infection or occurring at meal times perhaps due to obstruction. It may be persistent, either unilateral or bilateral, suggestive of a tumour, Sjörgen's syndrome, diabetes or alcoholism.

The minor salivary glands

Cysts

Diagnosis and presentation

Common sites include the lips, cheeks, floor of the mouth and palate. The cause is usually trauma, especially cheek or lip biting which may lead to stenosis or rupture of the duct and accumulation of saliva. They are common in children and young adolescents. The types include the mucous extravasation cyst and mucous retention cyst. In the former, mucus ruptures through the duct and pools in the adjacent connective tissue, there is no epithelial lining and the saliva is contained by flattened connective tissue. In the latter, mucus is still contained by the epithelium lining the duct, which swells to form an epithelial lined cyst (Fig. 16.1).

Signs and symptoms

These cysts usually present as painless, smooth, bluish swellings containing fluid. At intervals they burst, discharging their contents, but if untreated they heal and form again. In the floor of the mouth, a cyst may grow to a considerable size and is called a ranula.

Cysts treatment

Mucocele

Treatment involves delicate enucleation. An incision is made by drawing a scalpel blade lightly over the swelling and through the mucosa for a short distance beyond the lesion on each side. Alternatively an elliptical incision can be made to reduce the chance of rupture. The cyst is gently freed by blunt dissection and the gland concerned is also removed to prevent recurrence. Due to the fragile lining the lesion may burst during surgery. Other glands, seen in the wound, which may already be traumatised should be removed lest their ducts become blocked by scar tissue and give rise to new cysts. Primary closure is achieved by using superficial mucosal sutures.

Ranula

The ranula is more difficult to treat by enucleation. It may be treated with adequate marsupialisation. Following a lingual nerve block, the surface mucosa and roof of the cyst are excised. Care is taken to avoid damage to

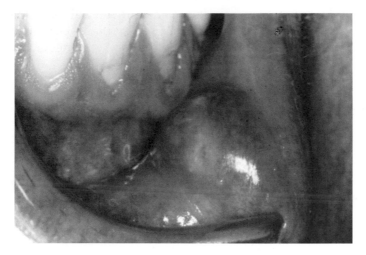

Fig. 16.1 Salivary mucocele of lower lip.

the submandibular duct and lingual nerve. The defect is packed with a Whitehead's varnish pack to allow epithelialisation from the base. Large cysts which are placed posteriorly (plunging), involving the sublingual gland, may necessitate gland removal.

Tumours

(See Chapter 15.) The commonest tumours include the locally invasive pleomorphic adenoma and the malignant adenoid cystic and mucoepidermoid carcinomas (Fig. 16.2).

Diagnosis

The pleomorphic adenoma occurs most frequently, with 70% occurring in the palate and the remainder in the upper lip or buccal mucosa. It presents as a painless nodule of rubbery consistency which may be fixed to either the overlying mucosa or the deeper structures. In the palate it is usually found to one side of the midline near the junction of hard and soft palate and may reach a considerable size.

The adenoid cystic and mucoepidermoid carcinomas may clinically resemble a pleomorphic adenoma but may display more rapid growth and ulceration of the surface mucosa.

Treatment

The pleomorphic adenoma is treated by excision with a wide margin of normal tissue to remove tumour cells lying outside the capsule. Large defects may require a skin or mucosal graft or rotational flaps or an oversown pack. Adenoid

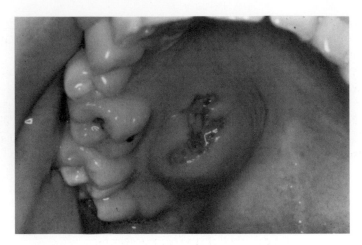

Fig. 16.2   Pleomorphic salivary adenoma in the palate. An incisional biopsy has been performed.

cystic carcinomas may spread far along the perineural lymphatics so that wide resection is necessary but occurrence is common. Radiotherapy is often used because a larger volume of tissue can be treated without mutilation. The mucoepidermoid carcinoma is usually successfully treated by surgery or radiotherapy.

The major salivary glands

The diseases of the major salivary glands requiring surgery include obstructions to salivary flow, infections and neoplasms.

Investigation of major salivary glands

Presentation and diagnosis

The clinician should record the presence of pain, swelling, altered salivary flow and a bad taste. The periodicity and duration of the swelling is often of great assistance in making a diagnosis. A subjective view of either an increase or decrease in salivary flow is made. However, this is difficult to confirm except by physiological methods of measurement which are not always easy to perform.

Probing the ducts can be carried out with care to dilate strictures. A stepwise increase in the size of the probes is used. Salivary flow rates can be recorded for the submandibular and parotid glands following initial milking of the ducts and glands.

Radiography

Radiographs in more than one plane are required. The submandibular gland can be examined using a lateral oblique projection of the mandible with occlusal views to show the duct. The parotid gland is seen on a postero-anterior view of the mandible with the central ray directed parallel to the ramus of the mandible or on a lateral radiograph, taken with the head extended to avoid superimposition of the vertebral column. An orthopantomogram may display both glands. Computerised tomography, magnetic resonance imaging and ultrasound may also be used.

Sialography

The indications for sialography include:

- Presence of a calculus, obstruction on eating
- Progressive enlargement – chronic, secondary to infection
- Visible and palpable swelling, lymphadenopathy, cystic lesion, tumour
- Recurrent sialadenitis
- Sjörgen's syndrome
- Post-trauma
- Pre-surgical assessment to determine the extent of a lesion and the appropriate site for biopsy
- Therapeutic reasons

The procedure involves passing a fine cannula into the duct orifice. A radiopaque contrast medium is used to outline the ductal architecture. The medium is introduced under pressure equal to about 70–90 mm of water. The procedure must not be used where there is acute infection in the gland or until radiographs have excluded the presence of a stone. Poorly calcified calculi may show as filling defects, stenosis as narrowing of the duct and tumours as an irregular filling pattern with areas of obliteration of the major and minor duct systems. The technique may be used with conventional radiographs and CT scans (see Fig. 16.3).

Scintiscan

This investigation has the advantage of examining all major salivary glands together. An intravenous injection of technetium is performed and the isotope is concentrated by the salivary glands. The head of the scanner picks up the radiation emissions producing a picture of the glands.

Biopsy

Minor salivary gland biopsies are performed where Sjogren's syndrome or other connective tissue disorders are suspected. Major gland biopsies can be performed. Fine needle aspiration is used to provide definitive diagnosis. It is

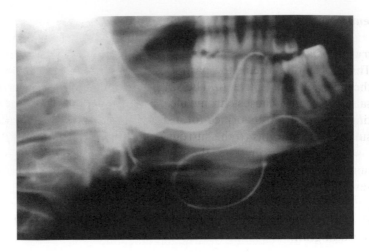

Fig. 16.3   Sialogram of submandibular salivary gland and duct.

indicated for determining whether a lesion is benign or malignant. It should indicate the tissue of origin and dictate the mode of treatment. The technique involves providing an aseptic field. A wide-bore needle, 18–20 gauge, is inserted into the gland. The target lesion is fixed between the index finger and thumb. The needle is aimed in the direction of the shortest distance to the lesion. The lesion is aspirated and the cellular contents deposited onto a glass slide and fixed immediately.

Obstructions to salivary flow

Aetiology

Aetiology may relate to stenosis of the duct papilla, sialadenitis, stricture of the duct, the presence of a salivary calculi or pressure on the duct from a nearby lesion.

Presentation

A recurrent painful swelling of the gland may be associated with meals or the sight of food. The swelling slowly goes down when the salivary stimulus is absent, only to recur at the next meal. Calculi can often be directly palpated using bimanual palpation.

Special investigations

These include radiography, sialography and judicious probing using lacrimal dilators.

Treatment of obstructions

Papillary stenosis

This more often affects the parotid papilla following trauma from dentures or the cusps of adjacent teeth. The submandibular duct may be affected where a salivary calculus causes chronic ulceration near the orifice. Treatment is by slitting the duct from its orifice for a short distance along its length and carefully suturing the margins to the surrounding mucosa.

A stricture remote from the papilla is not uncommon, though the cause if unrelated to trauma is not always clear. The stricture may be dilated using a series of urethral bougies along the duct, but if this fails the stoppage is bypassed by surgery to bring the duct into the mouth proximal to the obstruction. Parotid strictures may require part of the duct to be reconstructed using a mucosal graft.

Sialolithiasis

Siaoliths, calculi or stones are more common in the submandibular duct, almost three times more frequent than in the parotid.

Submandibular calculi

The common sites include the anterior two-thirds of the duct, the posterior third at the distal border of the mylohyoid muscle and within the gland itself. They are frequently seen as a yellow palpable swelling, tender when inflamed or infected, which can be felt on bimanual palpation intra- and extraorally. Their presence should be confirmed by radiography, usually a lower occlusal radiograph (Fig. 16.4).

When an acute infection is present first treat with antibiotics. Stones in the anterior two-thirds of the duct may be removed, under local anaesthesia, through an incision made parallel to the duct in the floor of the mouth. First the stone is accurately localised, by palpation. A suture is then passed deep to the duct and posterior to the stone and tied fairly tight to prevent the sialolith moving back towards the gland. The assistant should push up the floor of the mouth from below to improve access. Blunt dissection is performed to identify the calculus. The duct is incised and the stone removed. A false opening is required where the incision was made. Small incisions are usually left open but large ones may be partially closed and where necessary a drain is used to create a new orifice. Stimulation of saliva flow is important to keep the new opening patent.

Stones in the posterior part of the duct are more difficult to remove. Careful dissection must be performed to avoid damage to the lingual nerve, which crosses the duct in this region. Stones in the submandibular gland which cause symptoms are best treated by excising the gland. Complications of gland removal may include scarring, facial nerve palsy or lingual paraesthesia.

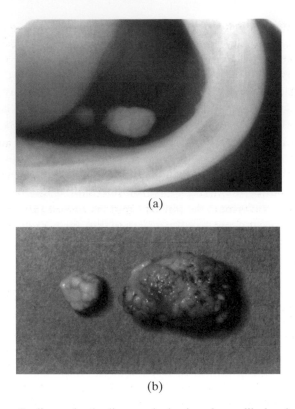

(a)

(b)

Fig. 16.4   Above: Radiograph of salivary calculus in submandibular duct. Below: Calculus after removal.

Parotid calculi

Parotid calculi may occur anywhere in the duct or gland. They are often poorly calcified and not easily seen on plain radiographs. Calculi in the duct can be removed through an intraoral approach, but the course of the duct through the buccinator muscle makes the operation difficult. Stones lodged in the gland usually produce minor symptoms and are best left untreated; others may have to be removed by excision of the part of the parotid gland in which they lie.

Lithotripsy

The destruction of calculi at other sites in the body (e.g. renal) by ultrasound is now routine practice and has had limited use for salivary calculi.

Infection

Acute sialadentis

The parotid is more commonly affected than the submandibular gland and the sublingual is rarely affected. Infection reaches the parotid gland through the duct. Predisposing factors include xerostomia, debilitation or disturbed function following abdominal surgery. The causal organism is usually staphylococcus. Acute submandibular sialadenitis is almost invariably associated with a salivary calculus, or stricture of the duct.

The gland is swollen, tender or painful and the patient is febrile. In the submandibular gland pus may be seen discharging from the duct. The floor of the mouth on the affected side is red and swollen. The parotid gland rarely discharges pus through the duct though the papilla is often inflamed and mumps should be excluded.

Patients with severe gland infections should be admitted to hospital. Initially vigorous antibiotic therapy is instituted and where indicated incision and drainage is performed. A salivary fistula is one of the complications. An incision a little way from the site of entry into the gland should avoid this. Oral hygiene should be carefully supervised. Where there is no obvious cause, a prolonged course of an antibacterial drug may be prescribed.

Chronic sialadenitis

Chronic sialadenitis commonly follows an acute attack and may result from prolonged obstruction to salivary flow. In the parotid gland it may be accompanied by sialectasis seen on sialography as dilatations of the ducts.

Treatment involves removal of any suspected underlying cause. Dilation of strictures to encourage salivary flow can be performed using lacrimal dilators. Careful use of antibiotic therapy may be required. If unsuccessful, excision of the submandibular gland is advised. Excision of the parotid gland is deferred whenever possible because of the danger to the facial nerve.

Tumours

Neoplasia usually presents as a non-tender swelling within the gland. The parotid gland is most often the site of tumours, the commonest of which is the pleomorphic adenoma, occurring ten times more often than in the submandibular gland. Benign lesions are treated by local excision. Wide excision of a pleomorphic adenoma should include daughter cells outside the capsule, which should reduce the likelihood of recurrence. Malignant lesions require radical surgery with facial nerve preservation where possible. However, the facial nerve may need to be sacrificed if involved in the tumour.

Presentation and diagnosis

Neoplasia is predominantly locally invasive or malignant in nature and differential diagnosis can be difficult.

Pleomorphic adenoma presents as a slowly enlarging, painless swelling. Sialography in the area shows obliteration of the normal duct structure.

Malignant tumours enlarge slowly with the additional symptom of pain. Growth involving the facial nerve leads to facial weakness. A diagnostic biopsy is contraindicated as it may lead to spread of the disease.

Treatment of tumours

The treatment of choice for lesions in the parotid is to excise the tumour with a wide margin of normal tissue, or in the submandibular gland to excise the whole gland.

Excision of the submandibular gland

A curved incision about 7.5 cm long is made in a crease of the neck about 2.5 cm below the lower border of the mandible to avoid the mandibular branch of the facial nerve (Fig. 16.5). The underlying fascia and platysma are divided. The facial vessels are detected and ligated. Blunt dissection or careful use of a finger separates the gland from the connective tissue. In long-standing chronic conditions dissection may be difficult due to fibrosis. The facial artery has to be ligated again on the posterior aspect of the gland. Superiorly the lingual nerve, which may be embedded in the capsule, is carefully dissected from the duct. The duct is ligated as near the mouth as possible and cut. If a stone is present check that it is in the excised gland. A vacuum drain is inserted to reduce post-operative swelling.

Surgery of the parotid gland

The approach to this gland is made through a preauricular incision extending from the temporal region to the angle of the mandible (Fig. 16.5). A facial flap is taken forward to expose the gland. The facial nerve which runs in the substance of the gland must be identified and dissected from the gland, every effort

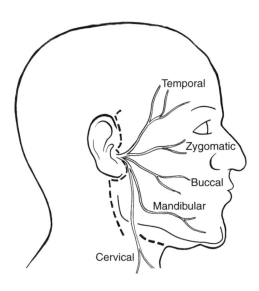

Fig. 16.5 Surgical approaches to major salivary glands. The approach to the parotid is an extended preauricular incision. The submandibular incision should be placed 2.5 cm below the lower border to avoid branches of the facial nerve.

being made to avoid production of facial weakness or paralysis. The auriculotemporal nerve may be damaged causing Frey's syndrome, a profuse and embarrassing facial sweating which the patient suffers when salivating.

Specific conditions

Mumps

Acute viral parotitis leads to salivary gland swelling, which commonly affects children under 15 years of age. Treatment is supportive, involving bedrest, analgesics and the encouragement of increased fluid intake.

Necrotising sialometaplasia

This condition presents at the junction of the hard and soft palate. It is commonly unilateral and may present as an extensive, deep, ragged-edged ulcer, which is usually painless. The condition is usually self-limiting over a period of 4 to 8 weeks. Difflam mouthwashes can be used if required.

Actinomycosis

In the parotid it may present in the acute or chronic form as an asymptomatic mass. Microbacterial assessment is required followed by the prescription of appropriate long-term antibiotics.

Tuberculosis

Presents as a firm non-tender swelling. It commonly affects the parotid gland but multiple gland involvement can occur.

Sarcoidosis

Sarcoidisis affects the parotid gland in 6% of cases. There is associated glandular enlargement and xerostomia.

Further reading

Cawson, R.A., Langdon, J.D. & Eveson, J.W. (1996) *Surgical Pathology of the Mouth and Jaws*. Wright, Oxford.

Soames, J.V. & Southam, J.C. (1993) *Oral Pathology*, 2nd edn. Oxford University Press, Oxford.

Chapter 17
The Temporomandibular Joint

- Pain dysfunction syndrome
- Osteoarthrosis
- Internal derangement
- Dislocation of the condyle
- Trismus
- Surgery
- Access to the joint

Surgery of the temporomandibular joint (TMJ) is seldom the treatment of choice. Disorders of the joint have a multifactorial aetiology and successful management lies in careful assessment of the joint, the muscles moving the mandible and the relationship between the mandible and the maxilla. Treatment involves co-operation between restorative dentists, orthodontists and oral surgeons. Only when conservative treatments have been extensively tried but have failed is surgery considered.

It is useful to consider the frequency with which disorders of the joint present as this emphasises the nature of the clinical problem. The commonest conditions are acute trauma including dislocation, osteoarthrosis (a degenerative condition), pain dysfunction syndrome and structural internal derangement. Less common are systemic diseases involving the joint, principally rheumatoid arthritis, but polyarthritic psoriasis and ankylosing spondylitis do sometimes involve the joint, though it is uncommon for local symptoms to be the patient's chief complaint or the reason for seeking treatment. Rarely, developmental abnormalities such as agenesis or hyperplasia of the condyle, suppurative infections and tumours occur.

Diagnosis

Diagnosis is made from the history, a careful examination of the joint, the muscles of mastication and of the occlusion, together with radiographs.

History

The history in acute trauma, dislocation and developmental abnormalities will strongly suggest the diagnosis. Internal derangement may result from trauma but this may be so insignificant (yawn or shout) that the patient is unaware of the event. Anterior displacement of the disc results in clicking and locking of the affected joint. By manipulation of the mandible, the patient can attain normal opening but with repeated trauma the disc becomes further displaced and the patient presents complaining of persistent restricted opening (closed lock). Pain due to secondary muscle spasm occurs late in the progress of the disorder.

Where there is an increased load on the joint due to bruxism or a deficient occlusion the pain dysfunction syndrome may result. The patient complains of a click, pain and trismus. The click may resolve as the condition progresses as jaw opening is limited by muscle pain. Resolution of symptoms occurs when the increased loading (e.g. bruxism) ceases but returns if causative factors reappear. The pain dysfunction syndrome is now recognised as a cause for headaches. The syndrome occurs in patients of 15–30 years of age and females present for treatment more commonly than males, although symptoms are found to be present equally in both sexes. Careful enquiry should be made as to any possible traumatic habits such as bruxism, clenching, nailbiting or overopening that might be contributing to the condition.

Should an increased load on the joint persist, degenerative changes may occur, resulting in osteoarthrosis, usually seen in patients over 40 years of age. The symptoms are pain and trismus worsening with increased use of the jaw. This may present towards the end of the day or in the morning if there is a tendency to night-time bruxism. Pain is limited to the area of the joint and crepitus is always present. Acute symptoms indicate erosion of the condyle or bony fossa while during repair and remodelling the patient has little discomfort or trismus though the crepitus persists.

Examination

The joint is examined by palpating the condyles just anterior to the tragus where its movements can be felt. Placing the little finger into the external auditory meatus allows palpation of the posterior aspect of the joint. The range of condylar movement is compared to the excursions of the mandible in opening and lateral movements. Tenderness to pressure is noted both over the condyle head and posterior to it when the mouth is open. Clicking and crepitus are important and are more easily heard with a stethoscope. The masseter muscle is palpated in the cheek while the body of temporalis is examined, with teeth clenched, in the temple region. Palpation along the anterior border of the ascending ramus towards the coronoid process may elicit tenderness in the temporalis tendon. Opening or lateral movement against pressure from the surgeon's hand produces pain in the lateral pterygoid muscle. Typically the masseter is painful in those who clench while temporalis is painful in bruxists.

The range of opening of the mouth and lateral movements performed should be measured for comparison of later progress. The minimal, normal opening is considered to be 35 mm in females, 40 mm in males. Measurement may be undertaken with a Willis or Vernier bite gauge. Lateral movements are measured by comparing the mandibular centre line with the maxilla and if less than 8 mm, are regarded as restricted. The teeth and occlusion are carefully charted and dentures assessed. Particularly important is whether centric relation and centric occlusion coincide. Any slide of the mandible from centric relation to centric occlusion and cuspal interferences on premolar or molar teeth are noted. Patients' occlusal habits such as clenching, protrusive movements or signs of bruxism such as attrition of the teeth, fractured cusps, ridging of the cheeks or scalloping of tongue are important.

Radiography

Satisfactory radiographs of the temporomandibular joint are difficult to take. Various views are used of which the transpharyngeal probably gives the best view of the condyle head. Interpretation also requires much experience as early changes are not easily identified or interpreted. Arthrography, where radio-opaque medium is injected into the joint space, gives an outline of the disc and shows displacement or perforation. Computerised tomography and magnetic resonance imaging techniques may aid diagnosis but in the commonest condition seen, the pain dysfunction syndrome, no changes are found by any imaging techniques.

Pain dysfunction syndrome

Clicking together with pain and limitation of movement constitute the temporomandibular joint pain dysfunction syndrome. It is associated with increased loading on the joint due to bruxism, clenching or occlusal interference. The onset of pain and trismus in many patients is related to muscle tenderness. Episodes of excessive bruxism and clenching, thought to be an emotional response, will lead to muscular pain. Clicking may be present only in the early stage of the syndrome and alone does not require treatment unless it causes the patient distress.

Treatment

A number of regimes have been used successfully. The simpler treatments that patients will find easy to follow are perhaps to be advocated. A full explanation of the aetiology and pathology of the condition may reassure the patient and allow them to modify damaging habits such as nail-biting or bruxism. The patients may only become aware of these habits after attention has been drawn to them and the use of these habits as stress relievers should not be underestimated. Resting the jaw by use of a soft diet and the use of anti-inflammatory drugs (Ibuprofen), if not contraindicated, will reduce pain.

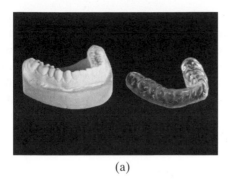
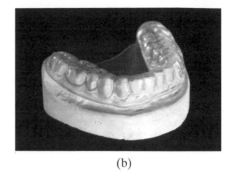

(a)   (b)

Fig. 17.1 Lower soft splint.

Exercises to normalise the pathway of opening and eliminate protrusive movements may help to reduce symptoms and prevent recurrence. To stop bruxism a soft splint over the lower teeth may help to break the habit (Fig. 17.1). If stress is an integral part of the problem recourse to antidepressant medication should be considered, while night sedation with benzodiazepines may also be useful. The patient's general medical practitioner should be advised and asked to assist in treatment. Occlusal interference if present may be eliminated by the use of a splint to provide balanced contact. If this proves curative a specialist restorative consultation should be sought.

Osteoarthrosis

This is a degenerative condition of the articulating surfaces of the joint. Whereas in an inflammatory lesion the pathological process starts in the synovium and thence affects the bone, current evidence suggests that in osteoarthrosis the primary disorder affects the subcondylar bone which becomes harder than normal, in turn affecting the overlying cartilage causing splitting, lipping and osteophytes. The disorder affecting the temperomandibular joint is probably secondary to trauma caused by overloading because of occlusal defects or bruxism. Epidemiological studies have shown degenerative lesions to be widespread among normal populations but patients only present for treatment when they experience pain possibly from a transient inflammatory episode.

Diagnosis

The symptoms are similar to those of the pain dysfunction syndrome, but the patients are usually over 40 years of age. The damaged joint surface produces a crunching sound (crepitus) on movement which can best be heard with a stethoscope. Erosions, when present, can sometimes be detected radiographically on the anterosuperior part of the condyle and its antagonistic area on the articular eminence.

Treatment

This is directed to relieving symptoms and prevention of further degeneration. Short-wave diathermy to the joint area and prescription of nonsteroidal anti-inflammatory drugs help the pain and trismus. Reduction of the load on the joint by occlusal rehabilitation should help to prevent the disease progressing. When the pathological changes are advanced, surgery may be indicated to remove the diseased condylar bone.

Internal derangement

Diagnosis of internal derangement may be difficult as the history is very similar to the pain dysfunction syndrome. Where the symptom of trismus fails to settle after the treatment outlined above, anterior displacement of the disc must be considered. This impedes the movement of the condyle resulting in limited opening.

Treatment

If the symptoms of pain and trismus are refractory to treatment and result in a significant impairment of daily activity such as eating and talking, the possibility of surgery should be considered.

Dislocation of the condyle

Dislocation of the condyle occurs usually in a forward direction over the eminentia articularis, and is often bilateral. The predisposing cause is laxness of the capsule and associated ligaments of the joint which allows excessive movement when opening the mouth wide as in yawning. Normal joints may be dislocated by a blow particularly while the mouth is open. Under a general anaesthetic dislocation can be caused by opening the mouth with a gag, or by downward pressure when extracting lower teeth, if the support to the jaw is inadequate.

Diagnosis

The patient complains of inability to bring the teeth together. In unilateral dislocation the midline of the mandible is deviated to the unaffected side. The dislocated condyle can be palpated in front of the eminentia articularis and radiographs confirm this position.

Treatment

If reduction is attempted immediately it can usually be achieved without sedation or a general anaesthetic. However, if some time has elapsed muscle spasm may make reduction difficult and relaxation of the muscles will be necessary either by the use of intravenous diazepam or a general anaesthetic. The operator places his thumbs (protected from the teeth by binding with gauze) over the external oblique line or retromolar fossa of the mandible on each side. The remaining fingers are cupped under the chin. While the thumbs press down, the fingers lift up the chin to slip the condyle head back over the eminentia.

Chronic recurrent dislocation

Where the capsule is very slack the condyle may dislocate several times a day. Many affected patients can reduce their mandibles at will, but others require it to be done for them. Surgery can be used for these chronic cases to restrict movement either by removing the eminetia, grafting bone over the eminetia to act as a stop, or by capsulorrhaphy, that is inserting fascial grafts or making a tuck in the capsule so that it is less lax. Alternatively the condyle head is excised.

Fractures of the condyle

These are discussed in Chapter 14.

Trismus

This is inability to open the mouth normally, and together with pain and clicking is one of the commonest symptoms associated with the temporomandibular joint and may be found in any of the conditions from which it suffers. As trismus is a symptom its cause should always be carefully sought, diagnosed and treated.

Persistent trismus may occur due to intra-articular fibrosis or bony ankylosis following trauma, infection or certain diseases such as rheumatoid arthritis. It may also be secondary to extra-articular fibrosis or scarring.

Intra-articular bony or fibrous ankylosis must be treated by surgery, either removal of the condyle (condylectomy) or cutting through the neck of the condyle (condylotomy). Trismus due to rheumatoid arthritis, ankylosing spondylitis or to extra-articular scarring may benefit from treatment with mechanical exercisers. Wooden spatulae in increasing numbers may be inserted between the teeth each day (Fig. 17.2). In more severe conditions the jaws are prised apart with Mason's gags used bilaterally under a general anaesthetic. Impressions are taken and a prop placed between the teeth until an exerciser can be fitted. Once a satisfactory opening (2.5 cm measured between the incisor teeth) has been obtained, this is maintained by using wooden spatulae for about 10 minutes each day for 6 months.

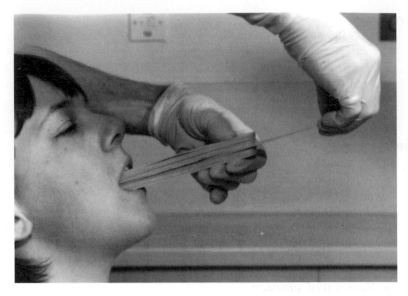

Fig. 17.2   Wooden spatulas in use to improve trismus.

Surgery

Surgical procedures are undertaken rarely but are indispensable in the management of ankylosis, growth disorders, recurrent dislocation and significant pathology including neoplasia. These disorders are uncommon but in the commoner lesions such as internal derangement the indications for TMJ surgery are less clear. The surgeon's task is to accurately interpret the symptoms reported by the patient, taking into account the success of non-surgical treatment, the disability suffered by the patient and the pathology underlying the condition. TMJ surgery may be indicated when:

- Symptoms are refractory to appropriate non-surgical treatment
- Pain is localised to the TMJ
- There is significant impairment of function
- There is pain on movement of the TMJ
- There is mechanical interference of TMJ function

Surgical procedures on the TMJ include:

- Arthrocentesis
- Arthroscopy
- Arthrotomy (open joint surgery)
- Condylotomy
- Joint replacement

Arthrocentesis

This is the simplest procedure involving lavage of the upper joint space via the insertion of two wide bore needles. This allows lavage of the joint with Ringers solution and some breakdown of adhesions. Its success in the treatment of anterior disc displacement has suggested that this may be due to reversible adhesions of the disc to the glenoid fossa.

Arthroscopy

Miniaturisation of instrumentation developed for use in larger joints has allowed procedures to be undertaken in a relatively non-invasive fashion. It has advantages over open joint surgery as it allows inspection of a surgically un-disturbed joint both at rest and in function. However, it only allows access to the upper joint space and is limited in the procedures and pathology it can be applied to. The procedures which can be performed are:

- Lavage
- Removal of adhesion
- Removal of damaged tissue
- Biopsy
- Plication to reposition displaced disc

Arthrotomy

Open joint surgery gives a complete range of surgical options from lavage, through disc plication to complete removal of the disc. In addition both upper and lower joint spaces may be entered. Care must be taken during the surgical approach to avoid damage to the facial nerve (Fig. 17.3).

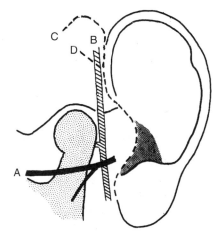

Fig. 17.3 Surgical approach to the temporomandibular joint. Note *A*, facial nerve, *B*, superficial temporal artery, *C*, line of preauricular incision, *D*, line of preauricular incision through the tragus.

Condylotomy

This is performed from an intraoral approach in a similar fashion to a vertical subsigmoid osteotomy (see Chapter 18). Osteotomising the condyle allows it to be repositioned anteriorly and inferiorly beneath the disc to improve function. Following the procedure there is usually a prolonged period of intermaxillary fixation to maintain the occlusion.

Total joint replacement

This is only indicated where there has been gross destruction of the joint architecture together with marked reduction in function. The surgical approach is via the preauricular incision (Fig. 17.3) together with a submandibular approach to allow wide exposure of the ascending ramus. Both the condylar head and the glenoid fossa components are replaced.

Access to the joint

The joint cavity is limited above by the zygomatic arch and posteriorly by the external auditory meatus. Surgery is made difficult by the facial nerve which passes through the parotid gland (in which it is quite deeply buried) about 2 cm below the zygomatic arch, and by the internal maxillary artery deep to the joint. The condyle is accessible only through an area about 2 cm^2 and may be approached by a preauricular incision made in front of the tragus and above the attachment of the lobe of the ear up to the zygomatic arch and then obliquely up and forward for 2 cm, or by a postauricular incision behind the ear which is then drawn forward to expose the joint (Fig. 17.3). The transverse facial and superficial temporal arteries may require ligation. The superior part of the parotid gland is drawn down, and the zygomatic arch cleared of the masseter. All stretching of the tissues to gain access is avoided lest it cause a facial nerve weakness.

Further reading

Dolwick, M.F. & Dimitroulis, G. (1994) Is there a role for temporomandibular joint surgery? *British Journal of Oral and Maxillofacial Surgery*, **32**, 307–13.

Jagger, R.G., Bates, J.F. & Kopp, S. (1994) *TMJ Dysfunction – the essentials*. Wright, Oxford.

Peterson, L.R., Ellis, E., Hupp, J.R. & Tucker, M.R. (1998) *Contemporary Oral and Maxillofacial Surgery*, 3rd edn. Mosby-Year Book, Missouri.

Chapter 18
Facial Deformity

- Symmetric facial deformity
- The cleft patient
- Orthognathic surgery
- Asymmetric facial deformity

Facial deformity may be the result of a variety of different causes including congenital disease such as cleft lip and palate, developmental abnormality, trauma and infection. Deformity may also occur, either as the direct result of a neoplastic disease or by its treatment either with surgery or radiotherapy.

Very occasionally deformity may occur with other acquired conditions which may affect facial growth such as juvenile rheumatoid arthritis (Still's disease), or it may occur after growth has ceased as with Paget's disease or other disturbances of bone metabolism such as fibrous dysplasia.

It is also important to remember that the face is comprised of both hard and soft tissue elements, and that deformity may derive from either element but very often one will impact on the other.

There is an obvious variation in facial form that gives us our individuality and ethnicity. Individuals who fall outside this acceptable range of variation may suffer from being labelled as either unattractive or ugly. This may cause the individual difficulties in social and sexual relationships and may deny certain employment opportunities. More severe facial deformity may cause social exclusion and can be associated with psychological problems.

This chapter aims to deal with the commoner types of facial deformity resulting from jaw growth disharmony, which often presents as malocclusion. The term 'dentofacial' deformity may be used to describe this problem. These problems usually result in symmetric facial deformity, and are treated jointly by the maxillofacial surgeon and orthodontist.

The commoner conditions resulting from a disease process are also addressed, such as cleft deformity. Asymmetric facial deformity may result from conditions such as hemifacial microsomia and condylar hyperplasia. Again collaboration between surgeon and orthodontist is required.

Assessment of facial deformity

History

The patient may identify problems as:

- Functional – difficulties associated with the bite, inability to chew or achieve incisor contact
- Aesthetic – problems of their appearance as perceived by them, although some patients may be embarrassed to discuss this

Patients are often referred by orthodontists who are unable to treat the underlying skeletal jaw disproportion by orthodontic means alone.

Examination

The patient is first examined by evaluation of the facial form, both from the profile and full face. It is helpful to divide the face into thirds (see Chapter 14). A full intraoral examination should include the state of the dentition as well as assessment of the occlusion. Poor dental health and hygiene are usually a contraindication to orthognathic surgery.

Radiographs

This includes a full radiographic assessment of the dentition including impacted and buried teeth, associated pathology including caries and periodontal problems. The lateral cephalostat provides invaluable information for both the surgeon and orthodontist to aid both diagnosis and treatment planning.

Study models

Study models should always be available at the joint consultation; anatomically articulated models are used in the surgical planning.

Photographic records

Photographic records are also extremely helpful in treatment planning as well as providing a clinical record. They should include both the face in profile and viewed from the front. Intraorally the occlusion should be shown from both sides and the front, and all photographs should be standardised and of good quality.

Special investigations

In some patients further information may be required both as part of the diagnosis and in planning treatment. Patients with asymmetric deformity may require special scans; these are discussed below in the relevant section.

Diagnosis

Symmetric facial deformity may be diagnosed and classified according to the facial types shown below. This classification is useful in prescribing the correct form of surgical correction to maximise successful and stable outcomes.

Symmetric facial deformity

Classification

The following is a useful classification of symmetric dentofacial deformity:

- Type A. Class III malocclusion due to either a large mandible or small maxilla (or both). The vertical height of the face is not increased. Treatment may involve moving the mandible posteriorly or the maxilla anteriorly (or both) (Fig. 18.1).

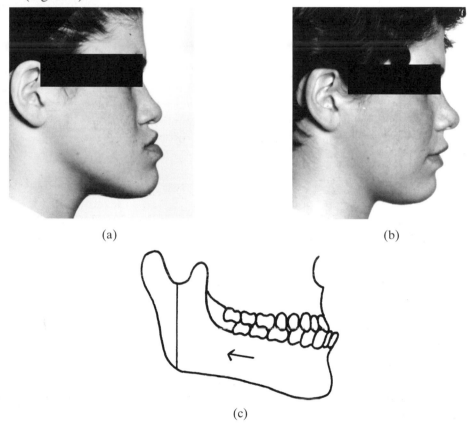

(a)   (b)

(c)

Fig. 18.1 Type A. Class III malocclusion. The mandible has been surgically repositioned posteriorly and the maxilla advanced: (a) pre-operative appearance (b) post-operative appearance (c) operative scheme.

- Type B. Class III malocclusion with an anterior open bite. This is due to either a large mandible or a small maxilla (or both). The vertical height of the face is increased. Treatment will always involve superior repositioning of the maxilla to reduce the increased vertical face height, together with posterior repositioning of the mandible (Fig. 18.2).
- Type C. Class II malocclusion with a deep overbite. This is due to a small mandible. The lower vertical face height is decreased. Treatment involves a mandibular advancement (Fig. 18.3).

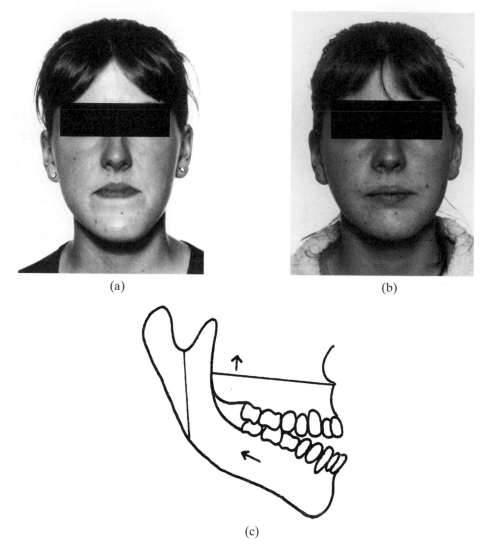

(a)   (b)

(c)

Fig. 18.2 Type B. Class III malocclusion with anterior open bite. Bimaxillary procedures have been used to superiorly reposition the maxilla and move the mandible posteriorly: (a) pre-operative appearance (b) post-operative appearance (c) operative scheme.

- Type D. Class II malocclusion with an anterior open bite. This is caused by an increased vertical growth of the maxilla in a downward direction. The mandible is of a normal size but has been rotated downwards and backwards by clockwise rotation due to the excess downward growth of the maxilla. Treatment involves superior repositioning of the maxilla following which the mandible autorotates anticlockwise to become normally positioned in relation to the face, and comes into a normal class I occlusion (Fig. 18.4).
- Type E. Class II with an anterior open bite. This is similar to Type D, however the mandible is small and the surgical correction requires a mandibular advancement together with superior repositioning of the maxilla (Fig. 18.5).

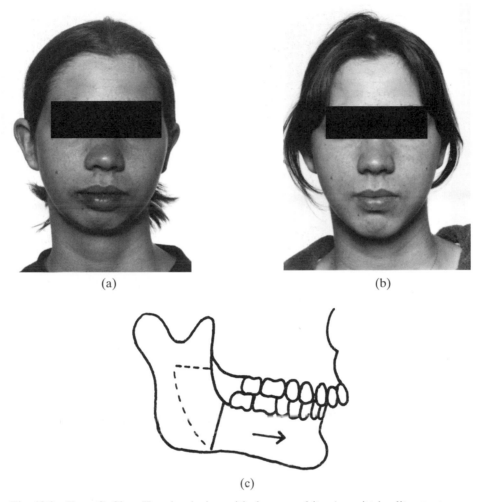

(a)

(b)

(c)

Fig. 18.3 Type C. Class II malocclusion with deep overbite. A sagittal split osteotomy has been used to advance the mandible: (a) pre-operative appearance (b) post-operative appearance (c) operative scheme.

Treatment planning

At a joint surgical and orthodontic appointment, the orthodontic treatment plan and provisional surgical correction are agreed between the patient and clinicians, and the anticipated outcome discussed. The orthodontic aspects are discussed below.

Final surgical plan

The final surgical plan is formulated following completion of the initial orthodontic phase of treatment. A new cephalostat showing the position of the teeth

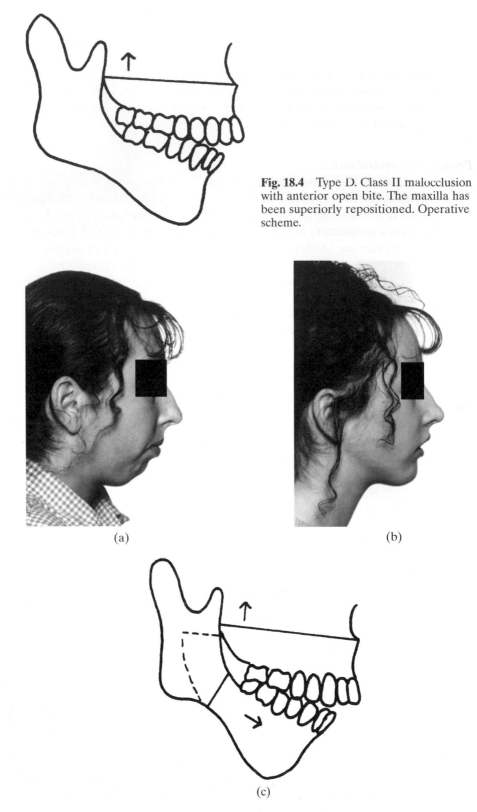

Fig. 18.4 Type D. Class II malocclusion with anterior open bite. The maxilla has been superiorly repositioned. Operative scheme.

(a)

(b)

(c)

Fig. 18.5 Type E. Class II malocclusion with anterior open bite and hypoplastic mandible. A bimaxillary procedure has been performed to superiorly reposition maxilla and advance the mandible: (a) pre-operative appearance (b) post-operative appearance (c) operative scheme.

following this orthodontic treatment is used to accurately plan the surgical procedure. This involves tracing the maxilla and mandible together with the dentition. A number of landmarks and references points are included to allow reproducible measurements.

Pre-surgical orthodontics

Orthodontic treatment is invariably required prior to undertaking surgery. This normally requires fixed appliances. The orthodontist carries out decompensation of the dentition, together with alignment and co-ordination of the dental arches to allow a satisfactory post-operative occlusion to be obtained. Decompensation involves moving teeth back to their normal alignment and angulations to the skeletal bases, often revealing the true skeletal problem (Fig. 18.6).

In type C cases it is recommended that flattening of the lower occlusal plane is not carried out pre-surgically. This allows the surgeon to produce a more satisfactory facial profile by lengthening the lower face. The immediate post-surgical occlusion achieved usually consists of 'heel and toe' contacts due to the uncorrected curvature of the lower occlusal plane. Post-surgically the orthodontist is able to extrude teeth into a satisfactory, stable and final occlusion.

Post-surgical orthodontics

This involves fine-tuning of tooth positions in most cases. In type C cases the patient should be aware that a considerable amount of orthodontic treatment is required to establish the final occlusal relationship.

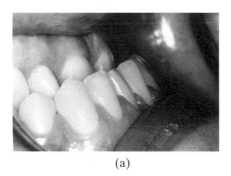

(a)

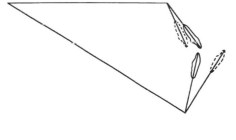

(b)

(c)

Fig. 18.6 Pre-surgical orthodontics: (a) Prior to treatment (b) Apparent worsening of the malocclusion (c) Decompensation to achieve ideal angulation of the teeth.

The cleft patient

Midface hypoplasia is commonly associated with cleft lip and palate patients. This is due largely to fibrosis from the primary repair disrupting normal maxillary growth. Thus maxillary advancement osteotomies are often required to establish a more normal facial profile and occlusion.

Alveolar bone grafting

Alveolar bone grafting is often carried out to re-establish continuity of the alveolus and allows eruption of the canine tooth.

Orthodontic considerations

Fixed appliance orthodontic therapy is required and will involve expansion of the contracted maxillary arch.

Special surgical considerations

Fibrosis following the primary surgery may impact on the ability of the surgeon to advance the maxilla into a satisfactory position. It is also important to take into account the patient's speech as nasal speech due to velopharyngeal incompetence may be exacerbated by maxillary advancement. Oronasal fistulae are often present and maxillary surgery may either produce or enlarge fistulae.

Orthognathic surgery

Orthognathic surgery is surgery to correct facial deformity and the associated malocclusion, (ortho = to straighten, gnath = jaws). The surgery involves carrying out bone cuts (osteotomies). Patients are managed jointly by the maxillofacial surgeon and orthodontist and close liaison and joint consultation are essential for optimum outcome of treatment.

Mandibular procedures

Sagittal split osteotomy

A sagittal split osteotomy is used to reposition the mandible anteriorly or posteriorly. The procedure is carried out via an intraoral incision and can be internally fixated with screws or plates. The disadvantage of the procedure is the relatively high incidence of permanent sensory loss to the lower lip as a result of injury to the inferior alveolar nerve (Fig. 18.7).

Vertical subsigmoid osteotomy

Vertical subsigmoid osteotomy is usually performed via an intraoral incision although previously an extraoral incision was employed. It is only used for pos-

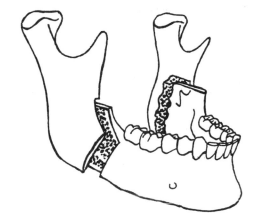

Fig. 18.7 Sagittal split osteotomy. The bone cuts can be rigidly fixed using plates and screws (see Chapter 14). Reproduced by kind permission of VU Press, Amsterdam.

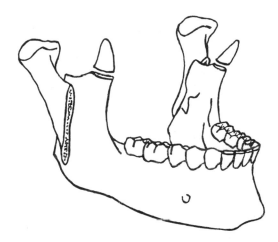

Fig. 18.8 Vertical subsigmoid osteotomy. It is difficult to rigidly fix the bone cuts when performed intraorally. IMF must be employed (see Chapter 14). Reproduced by kind permission of VU Press, Amsterdam.

terior repositioning of the mandible, and for minor mandibular asymmetries. It carries a low risk of injury to the mandibular neurovascular bundle. The major disadvantage of the procedure is that internal fixation cannot be applied when the procedure is carried out intraorally and thus intermaxillary fixation is required (Fig. 18.8).

Genioplasty

Genioplasty has no effect on the occlusion but is used to adjust the facial appearance by reduction or augmentation of the chin depth and prominence. It can be used to achieve chin symmetry and is performed via an incision in the lower labial sulcus.

Maxillary procedures

Le Fort I osteotomy

The position of the maxilla can be altered in all dimensions except posteriorly. It is performed via an intraoral incision and disarticulation of the maxilla from the facial skeleton is achieved by a series of bone cuts.

High Le Fort I osteotomy

The height of the bony incision can be raised to give more prominence to the mid part of the face following anterior movements (Fig. 18.9).

Maxillomalar advancement

Maxillomalar advancement is used to improve deficient prominence in the region of the cheekbones.

Le Fort II and Le Fort III osteotomy

These follow the fracture lines following facial trauma described by Le Fort (Chapter 14). They are performed less commonly and are used mainly to treat craniofacial abnormalities such as Treacher-Collins syndrome.

Segmental surgery is rarely required and indeed is a reflection of poor liaison between orthodontist and surgeon. Such surgery is often associated with poor outcome both in terms of the final facial appearance and iatrogenic periodontal problems or dental damage.

Internal fixation can be used to avoid the need for intermaxillary fixation in most cases apart from those patients undergoing an intraoral vertical subsigmoid osteotomy. Intermaxillary fixation if required is effected by means of the fixed orthodontic appliance.

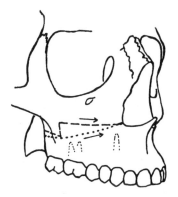

Fig. 18.9   Le Fort I osteotomy. Once mobilised the maxilla can be moved anteriorly, upwards and downwards. Reproduced by kind permission of VU Press, Amsterdam.

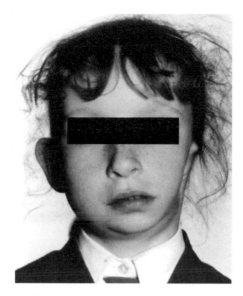

Fig. 18.10   Hemifacial microsomia.

Asymmetric facial deformity

Complete symmetry rarely (if ever) exists in nature and therefore asymmetric facial deformity may exist in a mild form in most individuals and may involve simply a lack of coincidence between the facial and dental midlines. Some individuals have a problem of sufficient magnitude to place them outside the range of normal variation, and often have an underlying pathology.

Individuals with asymmetric facial deformity often require special investigations to aid both diagnosis and eventual treatment planning, such as 3D imaging and the use of 3D models. If condylar hyperplasia is suspected then Technetium isotope scans may be employed to define if the condylar growth centre is still active prior to embarking on surgical correction.

Hemifacial microsomia

Hemifacial microsomia is a condition in which derivatives of the first branchial arch are incomplete or deficient. The ear is usually affected together with shortening of the mandibular ramus and varying degrees of abnormality of the temporomandibular joint. Surgical correction is complex and involves collaboration between the maxillofacial surgeon, orthodontist and facial prosthetist. Surgery will involve levelling of the occlusal cant due to the ramus shortening, and reconstructive surgery to restore facial symmetry (Fig. 18.10).

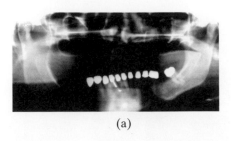

(a)

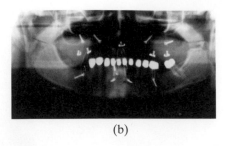

(b)

Fig. 18.11   Condylar hyperplasia: (a) The occlusal cant can be clearly seen. The mandibular midline has shifted to the left. (b) A unilateral mandibular osteotomy has been performed on the right. The patient was edentulous in the upper jaw.

Condylar hyperplasia

Condylar hyperplasia arises either when the condylar growth centre is reactivated after cessation of normal growth or when unequal activity during normal growth produces mandibular asymmetry. Correction may involve osteotomies of both the maxilla and mandible to correct occlusal cants and may also require pre-surgical orthodontiocs (Fig. 18.11).

Further reading

Tuinzing D.B., Greebe, R.B., Dorenbos, J. & van der Kwast, W.A.M. (1993) *Surgical Orthodontics – Diagnosis and Treatment*. VU University Press, Amsterdam.

Index